# Hospice and Palliative Care

# Jones and Bartlett Series in Oncology

*A Clinical Guide to Cancer Nursing: A Companion to Cancer Nursing,*
Groenwald/Frogge/Goodman/Yarbro

*Biotherapy: A Comprehensive Overview,* Rieger

*Bone Marrow Transplantation: Administrative Strategies and Clinical
Concerns,* Buchsel/Whedon

*Bone Marrow Transplantation: Principles, Practice, and Nursing Insights,
Second Edition,* Whedon

*Oncology Nursing Society's Building a Legacy: Voices of Oncology Nurses,*
Nevidjon

*Cancer and HIV Clinical Nutrition Pocket Guide,* Wilkes

*Cancer Chemotherapy: A Nursing Process Approach, Second Edition,*
Barton Burke/Wilkes/Ingwersen

*Cancer Nursing: Principles and Practice, Third Edition,*
Groenwald/Frogge/Goodman/Yarbro

*Cancer Pain Management, Second Edition,* McGuire/Yarbro/Ferrell

*Cancer Symptom Management,* Groenwald/Frogge/Goodman/Yarbro

*Chemotherapy Care Plans: Designs for Nursing Care,*
Barton Burke/Wilkes/Ingwersen

*Comprehensive Cancer Nursing Review, Second Edition,*
Groenwald/Frogge/Goodman/Yarbro

*Contemporary Issues in Breast Cancer,* Hassey Dow

*Handbook of Oncology Nursing, Second Edition,* Gross/Johnson

*Hospice and Palliative Care: Concepts and Practice,*
Sheehan/Forman

*Oncology Nursing Society's Instruments for Clinical Nursing Research, Second
Edition,* Frank-Stromborg

*Memory Bank for Chemotherapy, Second Edition,* Preston/Wilfinger

*Oncogenes, Second Edition,* Cooper

*Oncology Nursing Drug Reference,* Wilkes/Ingwerson/Barton Burke

*Oncology Nursing Homecare Handbook,* Barton Burke

*Oncology Nursing in the Ambulatory Setting,* Buchsel/Yarbro

*Oncology Nursing Society's Suffering,* Ferrell

# ❖ Hospice and Palliative Care

*Concepts and Practice*

*Edited by*

## DENICE C. SHEEHAN, RN, MSN, CRNH
## WALTER B. FORMAN, MD, FACP, CMD

JONES AND BARTLETT PUBLISHERS
*Sudbury, Massachusetts*

Boston          London          Singapore

*Editorial, Sales, and Customer Service Offices*
Jones and Bartlett Publishers
40 Tall Pine Drive
Sudbury, MA 01776
1-800-832-0034
508-443-5000

Jones and Bartlett Publishers International
Barb House, Barb Mews
London W6 7PA
UK

**Library of Congress Cataloging-in-Publication Data**

Hospice and palliative care : concepts and practice / [edited by]
   Denice C. Sheehan, Walter B. Forman.
      p.   cm.
   Includes bibliographical references and index.
   ISBN 0–86720–737–X
   1. Hospice care.  2. Palliative care.  3. Hospice care—United
States.  I. Sheehan, Denice C.  II. Forman, Walter B.
    [DNLM:  1. Hospice Care.  2. Palliative Care.  WB 310 H828 1996]
   R726.8.H653  1996
   362. 1'75—dc20
   DNLM/DLC
   for Library of Congress                       96–3660
                                          CIP

Printed in the United States of America

00  99  98  97  96    10  9  8  7  6  5  4  3  2  1

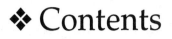

# ❖ Contents

*Foreword*     *vii*

*Preface*     *ix*

*Contributors*     *xiii*

**Part I**      **Introduction to Hospice**

1   The Historical Development of Hospice
    and Palliative Care     1
    DAVID A. BENNAHUM

2   The Referral Process and Reimbursement     11
    JUNE VERMILLON

3   The Interdisciplinary Team     21
    JEANNE M. MARTINEZ

4   The Core Team     31
    GARY A. JOHANSON
    INES V. JOHANSON

5   Additional Team Members     41
    LISA SZCZEPANIAK

6   Hospice Care Settings     51
    BETTY L. SCHMOLL
    CAROL E. DIXON

7   Quality Care in Hospice     61
    BETTY L. SCHMOLL
    CAROL E. DIXON

**Part II**      **Common Challenges Faced by the Team**

8   Pain Management in the Cancer Patient     71
    WALTER B. FORMAN
    DENICE C. SHEEHAN

9 Symptom Management 83
WALTER B. FORMAN
DENICE C. SHEEHAN

10 Common Questions and Concerns 99
DENICE C. SHEEHAN

11 Death Education: Teaching Staff, Patients, and Families
about the Dying Process 107
LAUREN R. ZEEFE

12 Ethical Issues in Hospice Care 115
DAVID BARNARD

13 Support Groups for Hospice Staff 131
LEONARD J. ZAMBORSKY

Part III Future of Hospice

14 Inclusion in American Health Care 139
JOHN J. MAHONEY

15 International Update 147
JOHN J. MAHONEY

16 Hospice and Palliative Care in Academia 151
WALTER B. FORMAN
DENICE C. SHEEHAN

17 Hospice Research 167
BETTY ROLLING FERRELL
BRANDI FUNK

Appendix I Assessment Tools 177

Appendix II Pain Diary 187

Appendix III Resources 191

Index 197

# ❖ Foreword

These are challenging times filled with great changes for hospice and palliative care. Since its establishment in the United Kingdom in the 1960s, hospice has been an exciting, innovative means of delivering a very different package of health care. No other attempt has been made to meet the patient's and caregiver's total needs in such a way as they have been met in hospice. Although it is sometimes difficult to explain and is often misunderstood, hospice has continued to deliver care of the highest quality in a changing health care sector. However, this evolving health care environment has placed new demands on hospice and its providers. Palliative care, traditionally delivered in an inspired, intuitive, but unplanned way, must now answer to formalized standards and heightened expectations.

This book, then, is a timely one. In tracing the development, success, and current dilemmas of hospice and attempting to predict its future, this book performs a valuable service to those wishing to know more about the process of hospice and its direction. In this readable book, one has a real sense that the contributors have grasped the issues around the provision of care, the recruitment of staff, symptom management, and the ethical issues that engage all in palliative care. In their well-referenced chapters they have managed to communicate their identity with and understanding of these issues.

I believe that in order for hospice to go forward, nurses and other members of the interdisciplinary team must be well supported, well managed, and free to express themselve Palliative care needs staff who will ask "why" without any fear of doing so. Without this ability to query the status quo, staff as independent and alive practitioners will disappear and quality palliative care will deteriorate. Quality of service is measured by the interaction between an individual staff member and an individual patient. If this is unsuccessful, the entire service is unsuccessful.

The late Robert Tiffany, director of nursing of Royal Marsden Hospital, once outlined five qualities that he thought paramount for any budding nurse: humor, honesty, heart, head, and humility. I believe these qualities are necessary for any practitioner contemplating palliative care. Certainly one should be able to provide compassionate care, but the helping hand should always be connected to a thinking brain. The chapters here on quality approaches and the need for continued research in palliative care reinforce the importance of critically evaluating clinical and organizational effectiveness, and the need for sensitivity when conducting research with this vulnerable group.

It is important that palliative care, arguably the most exciting development in medical care in the late twentieth century, not only continue to develop, but also be perceived by the public as a necessary, growing service. This book will provide a benchmark, a sense of reference for those involved, and also an introduction to those who seek to know more.

> Mr. Andrew Knight
> Chief Nurse
> St. Christopher's Hospice
> Sydenham, London
> England

# ❖ Preface

The rapidly evolving field of hospice and palliative care lacks easily accessible materials describing the essential elements necessary to initiate viable hospice and palliative care programs. Much of the available information deals with countries other than the United States. As palliative care clinicians and educators, we are keenly aware of this lack of information. This book begins to fill this void. The scope of hospice and palliative care, which encompasses many diseases, age groups, and humanistic issues, demanded that we provide the reader with an overall introduction to the concepts and practice involved in the care of these individuals. For the reader who wishes to explore each area in more depth, we have included additional references at the end of each chapter. We have emphasized the role of Medicare guidelines in directing hospice care, the role of the interdisciplinary team, the questions and concerns that we have experienced working in the field, and organizing and teaching care of the terminally ill. We hope this book will stimulate other health care workers to become involved in this relatively new, exciting field of health care.

Several terms in this book need clarification. *Family* refers to relatives and others who are important to the individual. The *interdisciplinary team* includes the individual and family as well as health care workers. We have attempted to separate the terms palliative care and hospice, although they are sometimes used interchangeably in the literature. The World Health Organization suggests the following definition for palliative care:

> Palliative care is the active total care of patients whose disease is not responsive to curative treatment. Control of pain, of other symptoms, and of psychological, social and spiritual problems is paramount. The goal of palliative care is achievement of the best possible quality of life for patients and their families. It affirms life and regards dying as a normal process. Palliative care neither hastens nor postpones death. It emphasizes relief from pain and other distressing symptoms, integrates the physical, psychological and spiritual aspects of patient care, offers a support system to help the patient live as actively as possible until death and a support system to help the family cope during the patient's illness and in their own bereavement.[1]

We define *palliative care* to include palliative medicine (the physician arm), palliative nursing, and other health care workers who care for the terminally ill and their families. *Hospice care* is that portion of palliative care which is predominantly provided in the home and in the growing number of hospice residential facilities. The National Hospice Organization offers the following definition of hospice:

> Hospice provides support and care for persons in the last phases of incurable disease so that they may live as fully and comfortably as possible. Hospice recognizes dying as part of the normal process of living and focuses on maintaining the quality of remaining life. Hospice affirms life and neither hastens nor postpones death. Hospice exists in the hope and belief that through appropriate care, and the promotion of a caring community sensitive to their needs, patients and their families may be free to attain a degree of mental and spiritual preparation for death that is satisfactory to them.[2]

This text is a shared work. We were pleased and honored by our coauthors as they each agreed with an energetic "yes" to our requests to join us in this endeavor. It is with sincere respect and appreciation that we acknowledge their work. We wanted the writing to reflect the interdisciplinary roles inherent in hospice and palliative care as well as the individuality of each of the writers. Therefore, we have not imposed a consistency of style on their writing, but rather left them to express their thoughts in their own ways. We believe this has enriched the book. We also wish to express our sincere thanks to those who have so graciously given of their time, energy, and expertise as reviewers, both formally and informally. The following people deserve special thanks: Galen Miller and Glenn Gillen of the National Hospice Organization, Kathy Ryan, Connie Krug, Georgette Frate-Mikus, Dave Vogan, Carol Patacca, Paul and Barbara Kopchak, Jane Bigler, and Bruce Agneberg. We would also like to thank Jan Wall, Suzanne Crane, Mary Sanger, and Kelly Bechen for providing guidance and polish for this project. We are especially grateful to our spouses, Rick and Beverly, who listened to our ideas and supported our work.

Others have influenced our work as mentors. Denice would like to thank Elizabeth Pitorak for sharing her visions and high standards of care, Polly Puzder for her support and insights, Pat Kelley and Connie McPeak for stimulating discussions about metaphors and spiritual growth, and the nursing faculty at Ursuline College for supporting palliative nursing in the curriculum.

Walter would like to thank Robert Twycross, who introduced him to the many facets of palliative medicine, Balfour Mount for his willingness to share his experiences, Andrew Hoy for sharing his knowledge about how a community-based program is developed and maintained, and Rod McLeod for stimulating his interest in the innovative ways to teach palliative medicine.

He especially wishes to thank the faculty and house staff at Case Western Reserve University during the 1960s and 1970s who were responsible for developing his interest in the understanding, teaching and caring for people who were faced with a life-threatening illness.

Finally, we would like to dedicate this book to our colleagues who wish to learn more about hospice and palliative care. It is our hope that many people will benefit from a knowledgeable interdisciplinary health care team working to relieve those who suffer.

## ❖ References

1. World Health Organization. *Cancer Pain Relief and Palliative Care.* Technical Report Series 804. Geneva: World Health Organization, 1990.
2. National Hospice Organization. *Standards of a Hospice Program of Care.* Arlington, VA: National Hospice Organization, 1993.

# ❖ Contributors

David Barnard, PhD
Professor and Chairman,
   Department of Humanities
The Pennsylvania State University
   College of Medicine
Hershey, Pennsylvania

David A. Bennahum, MD
Professor of Medicine and Family
   and Community Medicine
University of New Mexico
Albuquerque, New Mexico

Carol E. Dixon, RN, MS
Vice President and Chief
   Operating Officer
Hospice of Dayton, Inc.
Dayton, Ohio

Betty Rolling Ferrell, PhD, FAAN
Associate Research Scientist
City of Hope National Medical Center
Duarte, California

Walter B. Forman, MD, FACP, CMD
Associate Chief of Staff,
   Geriatrics/Extended Care
Albuquerque Veterans
   Administration Medical Center
Professor, Medicine and Geriatrics
University of New Mexico
   School of Medicine
Albuquerque, New Mexico

Brandi Funk, RN, BSN
Research Specialist
City of Hope National Medical Center
Duarte, California

Gary A. Johanson, MD
Director, Palliative Care Service
Hematology Oncology Group
Santa Rosa, California

Ines V. Johanson, RN, CRNH
Director of Nursing
National Home Care Nursing
   and Hospice
Santa Rosa, California

Andrew Knight, RGN
Chief Nurse
St. Christopher's Hospice
Sydenham, London
England

John J. Mahoney
President
National Hospice Organization
Arlington, Virginia

Jeanne M. Martinez, RN, MPH
Coordinator
The Center for Palliative Medicine
   Education and Research
Northwestern Memorial Hospital
Chicago, Illinois

Betty L. Schmoll, RN, MS
President and CEO
Hospice of Dayton, Inc.
Dayton, Ohio

Denice C. Sheehan, RN, MSN, CRNH
Instructor, Division of Nursing
Ursuline College
Pepper Pike, Ohio

Lisa Szczepaniak, RN, BSN, CRNH
Hospice Nurse Clinician
Hospice of the Western Reserve
Cleveland, Ohio

June Vermillon, RN, BSN
Director, Hospice Services
Presbyterian Home Healthcare
Albuquerque, New Mexico

Leonard J. Zamborsky, PhD, MA,
    MDiv
Psychologist, private practice
Pastor, St. Louis Church
Cleveland Heights, Ohio

Lauren R. Zeefe, MEd, LPC
Certified Grief Counselor
    and Death Educator
Counselor
Ursuline College
Pepper Pike, Ohio

## ❖ Chapter 1

# The Historical Development of Hospice and Palliative Care

DAVID A. BENNAHUM

The care of suffering and dying patients is part of human history. In the past quarter of a century, however, we have seen a revolution in the care of terminally ill patients and those in pain. This is the result of a number of individuals whose critical thinking has reshaped contemporary views of death. In 1963, Jessica Mitford satirized American attitudes towards death in her mordant book (later produced as a film), *The American Way of Death*.[1] Philippe Aries, in his extraordinary 1981 book, *The Hour of Our Death*, examined how Western civilization had come to conceal death in the late nineteenth and twentieth centuries as the Victorians had concealed sexuality in the last century.[2]

As early as 1914 Justice Cardoza asserted the right of individuals to refuse care in a disserting U.S. Supreme Court decision. However, it took a legal and ethical evolution to confirm that patients had the right to be informed about their care, and that health professionals and hospitals were accountable for that care. It was this belated recognition that was confirmed by the United States Congress in 1991 in the Danforth Amendment. This law requires that patients admitted to health care facilities receiving federal funds be informed of their right to refuse care and to have advanced directives for health care.* In addition, a better understanding of pain control and a variety of methods for achieving this end have developed. Despite this landmark legislation, as we will see later in this chapter the work of two women physicians, Elisabeth Kubler-Ross and Dame Cicely Saunders, perhaps more than anything else, began to change the way society and health professionals perceived terminal disease, death, and dying.[3]

## ❖ The Historical Roots of Hospice

Among the Greeks in Homeric times (8th century B.C.), all strangers without exception were regarded as being under the protection of Zeus Xenios, the god of strangers and suppliants. A wanderer would be treated as a guest and offered food, shelter, clothing, and gifts. Violation of the duties of hospitality were likely to provoke the wrath of the gods.

---

*The Danforth Amendment required that as of 1991 all patients admitted to health care facilities receiving federal aid be advised of their right to refuse care.

In the Greek culture, patients who were not cured by an itinerant physician, the Iatros, could seek care at a temple to Aesculepius, the god of medicine. Here they would spend the night in the temple precincts "incubating" with the god. In the morning the priests of Aesculepius would interpret the patients' dreams. Over time these temples became places where medicine was taught.[4]

In Roman times the custom of private hospitality was codified and legally defined. Host is derived from the root *hospes*. Ties between a guest and a host, meaning the person who receives or entertains, were confirmed by the clasping of hands and the exchange of a written agreement, the *tabula hospitalis*. This sacred contract in the name of the god Jupiter Hospitalis developed into a practice whereby the Roman state appointed citizens of foreign states, called the Public Hospitium, to protect Romans abroad.[5] Hospice derives from the Latin *hospitium*, meaning entertainment, hospitality, lodging, or inn.[6] Thus the place where a guest was received evolved into *hospital* for the temporarily sick and *hospice* as a place for the permanent residence for poor, infirm, crippled, insane, and incurable people. Other related words such as hostel, hotel, host, and hostess also were derived from *hospitium*.

The first hospitals appeared on the periphery of the Roman Empire and were military hospitals that served the legions garrisoned on the frontier.[7] By the fourth century, first in Byzantium and later in Rome under the impetus of early Christianity, rudimentary hospitals and hospices began to appear that welcomed travelers and cared for the sick. Dame Cicely Saunders, the founder of St. Christopher's Hospice, points out that, "This was a radically different approach to the Hippocratic tradition in which a doctor did not treat the incurably sick or terminally ill. It was thought unethical to treat a patient with a deadly disease, for in so doing the doctor risked paying the penalty awaiting those mortals who challenged nature and the gods."[8] In the Middle Ages (476–1453 A.D.) hospices sprang up along routes of commerce and pilgrimage, the most famous being those at alpine passes maintained by the order of St. Bernard. As a response to the Crusades, the order of Knights Hospitalers established hospitals in Europe and the Middle East along the Crusader and pilgrimage routes. Leprosy spread widely during the Middle Ages, but is not found in skeletal remains prior to the fourth century A.D.[9] The leprosy described in the Bible is probably a group of skin diseases such as psoriasis. In response to the medieval epidemic of leprosy, houses dedicated to Lazarus, who is mentioned as healed by Christ in the Roman Book of St. Luke, sprang up near more than 4,000 towns and cities in France and Germany.

It is important to remember that both ancient India and Egypt had institutions that had some of the attributes of hospitals. Egypt, as early as 2500 B.C., had a highly organized system of medical education and health care as is seen in such documents as the *Smith Papyrus*.

According to Indian literature in the sixth century B.C., Buddha appointed a physician for every ten villages and built hospitals for the crippled and the poor; his son built shelters for diseased and pregnant women. Hospitals existed in Ceylon as early as 437 B.C. The most outstanding of the early hospitals in India were the eighteen built by King Asoka (273–232 B.C.). These are historically significant because of characteristics similar to those of the modern hospital (or hospice). The attendants were ordered to give gentle care to the sick, furnish them with fresh fruits and vegetables, prepare medicines, give massages, and keep their own persons clean. Hindu physicians . . . were required to take daily baths, keep their hair and nails short, wear white clothes, and promise to respect the confidence of their patients.[10]

Islam also played a prominent role in the institutional care of the sick, particularly the mentally ill, introducing the idea of humane care in special asylums.

As European cities began to grow in the Renaissance, (1300–1600 A.D.) the need for the care of indigent, old, and insane individuals became essential. Modeled on the leprosaria of the middle ages, hospices evolved that provided minimal shelter and food for this population.[11] In addition to leprosaria and hospices, another peculiar institution of the Renaissance was the foundling hospital, which acted as a population control system by accepting unwanted newborns, previously given to medieval monasteries and convents, where they often died of infection and neglect.[12] These institutions evolved into the hospitals of the eighteenth and nineteenth centuries whose high rates of infectious diseases resulted in horrendous mortality rates.[13]

The discovery of anesthesia in 1842 and Lord Lister's aseptic surgical technique together revolutionized medicine by the end of the nineteenth century.[14] Amputations could be performed and cancers resected without pain and with very little risk of infection. Western medicine had always been heroic; that is, advocating purges, cathartics, emetics, and bleeding to remove noxious humours as advocated by Galenic principles. The Idea of Progress, introduced by Sir Francis Bacon in his *Great Instauration of Knowledge* published in 1626, set the ground for the optimistic positivism and meliorism that often drives the care of patients to this day.[15] It has become difficult not to treat, for to do so is to threaten the almost universally held belief that science can only improve the human condition.

## ❖ The Modern History of Hospice

### *Dame Cicely Saunders*

It was in the setting of the exponential growth of Western medical science in a society that was paradoxically denying the inevitability of death that Elizabeth Kubler-Ross and Cicely Saunders were to make their extraordinary contributions. A number of institutions had recognized the need for humane care of the dying in the nineteenth century. Saunders, in her introduction to the *Oxford Textbook of Palliative Medicine*, notes that Jeanne Garnier in Lyons, France founded several hospices or Calvaires as early as 1842.[8] The Irish Sisters of Charity opened Our Lady's Hospice in Dublin in

1879 and St. Joseph's Hospice in East London in 1905, both for incurable or dying patients. Inspired by these examples, Calvary Hospital in New York was opened in 1899. Additionally, three Protestant homes for the dying had been opened in London by the turn of the century. These were the Frieden-shein Home of Rest, later St. Columbus Hospital in 1885; the Hostel of God that became Trinity Hospice in 1891; and St. Luke's Home for the Dying Poor established in 1893 to care for those dying of tuberculosis and cancer.[8]

Dame Cicely Saunders entered medical school at St. Thomas Hospital Medical School in London in 1951 after originally training as a nurse at the Nightingale School at St. Thomas Hospital. She had also finished a degree in philosophy, politics, and economics at Oxford and gained a diploma in Public Administration. From the beginning of her work as a nurse, Saunders seems to have recognized that cancer patients challenged the prevailing optimism of medicine. She credits her seven years as a volunteer nurse at St. Lukes beginning in 1948, and writes that "... the reading of its many full and lively reports by Dr. Howard Barrett, its founder, were major influences in the early planning of St. Christopher's Hospice,"[8] which she would help found in 1962. His turn-of-the-century records described patients and the benefits of good pain control. It was at St. Lukes that she came to understand the need for home care, family support, research, and education and that pain and symptom control were crucial. This lead her to spend an additional two years of fellowship studying pain control in the Department of Pharmacology at St. Mary's Medical School in London.

Having completed her medical studies in 1957, Saunders began working at St. Joseph's Hospital in Hackney, a working-class section of London. Here she began her work in the use of opioids to control pain in dying patients. On the basis of what she had learned at St. Lukes, she experimented with higher doses of opiates that were given in advance of pain and on a regular schedule. Through this she observed (as Kubler-Ross later would) that patients free of pain were only too eager to talk about their illness and that they benefited from the opportunity.[3] On the basis of her experiences Saunders wrote a series of insightful articles and developed a personal network of colleagues and friends. By 1967 she was able to raise enough money and persuade the National Health Service to give her sufficient support to design and build St. Christopher's Hospice in Sydenham on the outskirts of London. Her practical, patient-centered approach would have appealed to Thomas Sydenham, a great seventeenth century physician, known as the English Hippocrates who rebelled against the heroic treatments with emetics, cathartics, and bleeding of his time. On the basis of her remarkable preparation, Saunders was able to understand the complex interdisciplinary needs of cancer patients and formulate the following principles:

1. Death must be accepted.
2. The patient's total care must be managed by a skilled interdisciplinary team whose members communicate regularly with one another.
3. The common symptoms of terminal disease, especially the palliation of pain in all its aspects, need to be controlled effectively.

4. The patient and family as a single unit of care must be recognized.
5. An active home care program should be implemented.
6. An active program of bereavement care for the family after the death of the patient must be provided.
7. Research and education should be ongoing.[3]

## Elizabeth Kubler-Ross, M.D.

During the same period in which Saunders was doing her creative work in Great Britain, Kubler-Ross had spent a number of years interviewing dying patients. As a psychiatrist, she had found it very hard to find patients to interview because most physicians and nurses thought her interest morbid if not perverse. Persisting in her inquiry, she published *On Death and Dying* in 1969, for the first time creating a theoretical framework that described the psychological stages of dying as she perceived them.[16] The impact of Kubler-Ross's work on the popular and professional environment in the United States was crucial to the acceptance of hospice treatment as proposed by Saunders. The taboos and silence erected in the nineteenth and twentieth centuries had to be challenged before the idea of palliative care could be considered. Although some of Kubler-Ross's stages would prove to be less certain than she had proposed, the study of the dying process would now be acceptable if not downright fashionable. The prevailing positivism of American medicine continues, but it is now possible to challenge the melioristic assumption that the full thrust of treatment should be to extend life at all cost.

## Early Hospice in the United States and Canada

The work at St. Christopher's awakened the interest of physicians and nurses in the United States. As early as 1963, Saunders had been invited to lecture at the Yale University School of Medicine. There she met Florence Wald, then dean of the graduate school of nursing. In 1966 Wald invited Saunders back to present a workshop on hospice. This was the beginning of hospice in the United States. Florence Wald opened the New Haven hospice homecare component in 1974. The inpatient service opened in 1979 with Sylvia Lack as its first medical director. This created a new model that was able to demonstrate that Americans were comfortable with home care. This was confirmed by the Hospice of Marin near San Francisco, opened in 1976 and directed by Dr. William Lammers, that focused on home care and was largely sponsored and supported by lay workers and volunteers.

Another hospice directed by physician Balfour Mount opened at the Royal Victoria Hospital of McGill University in Montreal. This model demonstrated the value of the presence of a hospital-based palliative care service, especially in terms of research and education on pain control. It was Mount who first used the term *palliative care*. In 1977 the hospices of Marin and Yale sponsored the first major conference on care of the dying which attracted representatives from seventeen states.

On the basis of another model, that of an interdisciplinary palliative care group as developed at St. Luke's in New York, its proponents would argue that:

> Hospice care should be part of the mainstream of American Medicine and its institutions. Development of separate facilities for hospice care could be more costly and might result in the public perceiving hospices as another form of nursing home. Furthermore, hospital care should be influenced by the principles of hospice care; that is, caring and curing should be related. A hospice team or consultant in every teaching hospital would enable today's students and tomorrow's health care providers to observe hospice care as an integral part of treatment in the acute care setting."[3]

## *The Legislative Role in Hospice and Palliative Care*

In 1972 the United States Senate's Special Committee on Aging held hearings on "Death with Dignity."[17] Whereas at first hospice organizers sought to separate hospice from traditional hospital care (seeing hospital technology as preventing humane care of the dying), the government now became interested in incorporating hospice care into the work of traditional institutions. By the late 1970s, interest in the process of dying became widespread in the United States. Kubler-Ross' book had become well known and the subject of innumerable radio, television, and magazine discussions. In the late 1970s, the New Haven hospice program assisted in bringing together hospice advocates in North America. The meeting was held to establish guidelines for operational issues necessary to develop hospice programs. The meeting was successful and the National Hospice Organization was born. In 1983 the National Hospice Organization was able to persuade Congress to establish hospice benefits for Medicare beneficiaries. As might have been predicted for America, however, enthusiasm for palliative care of terminal illness led to the appearance of an eclectic mix of hospice programs. By 1985 there were more than 1,500 in the United States that ranged from home care to hospital care, and from professional palliative care teams to lay and volunteer workers.

The development of the hospice movement paralleled an increasing concern for the unnecessary prolongation of life. The 1976 Quinlan decision, permitting the removal of a ventilator from a comatose young woman, was followed by fifteen years of remarkable legal decisions and the evolution of biomedical ethics as a patient care discipline. Most recently, the 1991 Supreme court decision in the case of Nancy Cruzan affirmed the right of patients to have advanced directives and to refuse medical care. Interest in death and dying is now focused on the controversial issues of assisted suicide and euthanasia with forces polarized between the ideas of the right to die and the right to life movements. Contemporary palliative care advocates almost universally assert that if pain and suffering are relieved, then requests for assistance in dying are rarely made. Not all commentators agree with this opinion, especially as one moves from a consideration of the experience of cancer patients to that of terminal AIDS, end-stage renal disease, and severe, chronic depression.[18,19,20]

## ❖ The Contribution of Pharmacological Innovation

The distinguished British medical historian, Roy Porter, in his encyclopedia of the history of medicine published in 1993, points out that, "Pain is one of the more puzzling, and neglected, topics of the history of medicine . . . it is, however, central to the healer's art. Critics of high-tech modern medicine such as Ivan Illich have deplored this retreat from the head-on confrontation with pain. Such refusal to face reality, they allege, undermines self-management and personal control. He or she who cannot face pain will not be able to face death. Yet, as is amply shown by the liberal policy with morphine dosages followed in British hospices, the signs are that effective pain control can materially enhance the quality of life in the terminally sick. Successful pain management may be one of the more tangible and widespread, if less glamorous, triumphs of modern medicine."[21]

The *Smith Papyrus* mentions the "red shepenn," which seems to mean opium poppy, and small juglets in the form of opium poppy capsules were exported from Cyprus to Egypt as early as 1500 B.C. Before the time of the Greek war against Troy, approximately 1300 to 1200 B.C., there already existed a Minoan cult on the island of Crete, to the goddess of the poppy. There was a "tradition whereby opium was the active principle of Helen's famous Egyptian potion, *nepenthes,* which relieved the deepest sorrows."[7] Opium was always an ingredient of Theriac, the universal panacea first created by King Mithridates as an antidote to poison, and later enhanced by Nero's physician, Andromachus with up to sixty ingredients. Galen wrote a book on the subject and Theriac was in common use until the end of the nineteenth century. The Chinese would call it *te-ya-ka* and the great Hindu medical books of *Charaka* and *Sushruta* mention similar complex potents all of which probably contained opium.[7]

For the treatment of pain the Graeco-Roman physician had opium, wine, and the alkaloids of henbane, belladonna, black nightshade, and mandrake from which are derived hyoscyamine, atropine, and scopalamine. These were used both as poisons and analgesics.[22] A number of historians believe that there were other pain relievers; Hippocrates mentions a lost text, *On Drugs,* but these are unknown today. For the treatment of the podagra of gout, the Byzantine physician Alexander of Tralles (A.D. 525–605) recommended the emetic properties of the autumn crocus. In the nineteenth century colchicine was derived from that flower, and shown to be a specific anti-inflammatory agent for the pain and swelling of gout.[11]

Tea brewed from the bark of the willow tree, Salix alba, has been used to treat arthritis for generations. The Doctrine of Signatures states that the cure for many symptoms can be found in the place where the disease occurs.

For example, the pain of arthritis is often worse in swampy areas where the willow tree grows. The Reverend Edward Stone published a paper in the *Philosophical Transactions of the Royal Society* in 1763 advocating the use of willow bark in the treatment of arthritis and fever.[23] First the specific, salicin, was isolated from the willow and later acetylsalicylic was synthesized by Charles Gerhardt in 1853 in Strasbourg and introduced into clinical practice by Heinrich Dreser while working for the Bayer company in 1899.

The search for analgesic and antipyretic drugs led nineteenth century German chemists to examine coal tar and its derivatives, leading to the discovery of the analines, so important to the dye industry; phenols that were antiseptic; pyrazolines and thus antipyrine that were anti-inflammatory and analgesic. These researchers would eventually produce acetaminophen. The discovery of ACTH, the corticosteroids, and the nonsteroidal anti-inflammatory drugs (NSAIDs) after the Second World War would in turn enhance the ability of physicians and nurses to control pain.

America's greatest contribution to medicine, Crawford W. Long's demonstration in 1842 of the anesthetic properties of ether (later controversially claimed by Horace Wells and W.T.G. Morton), introduced painless surgery to the world.[11] A few years later, in 1853, C.G. Pravaz and Alexander Wood introduced the hypodermic syringe. Mid-century physicians were now able to inject the newly isolated opiates, morphine and heroin, as well as cocaine. The availability of anesthesia and opiates by syringe would soon be tested in the cauldron of the Civil War, initiating the modern era of anesthetic surgery, as well as the plague of intravenous addiction.[14]

## ❖ Summary

In his recent book, *How We Die,* Sherwin B. Nuland emphasizes the importance of hope to each and every patient.

> Hope lies not only in an expectation of cure or even of the remission of present distress. For dying patients, the hope of cure will always be ultimately false, and even the hope of relief too often turns to ashes. When my time comes, I will seek hope in the knowledge that insofar as possible I will not be allowed to suffer or be subjected to needless attempts to maintain my life; I will seek it in the certainty that I will not be abandoned to die alone; I am seeking it now, in the way I try to live my life, so that those who value what I am will have profited by my time on earth and be left with comforting recollections of what we have meant to each one another.[24]

The hospice movement was grounded in the belief of a few courageous pioneers that dying patients need not suffer alone and without respite. The discipline to study pain, dying, and death did not come easily, and has had to challenge the prevailing view that death is a failure of medicine and something to be hidden and avoided. Emerging from a religious impulse to comfort the sick, the care of the dying was greatly facilitated by research into pain management and a better understanding of the importance of symptom relief, be it thirst, hunger, inflammation, anxiety, depression, or pain. Surprisingly it has taken, and still takes, rigor, discipline, and objective observation, as well as compassion and competence to persuade health professionals and often patients, that death with dignity is not giving up; rather, it can be the proper completion of an individual life.

## ❖ References

1. Mitford, J. *The American Way of Death.* New York: Simon & Schuster, 1963.
2. Aries, P. *The Hour of Our Death.* New York: Alfred A. Knopf, 1981.
3. Torrens, P.R., ed. *Hospice Programs and Public Policy.* Chicago: American Hospital Publishing, American Hospital Association, 1985.
4. Edelstein, L. *Ancient Medicine.* Baltimore: Johns Hopkins University Press, 1967.
5. Encyclopaedia Britannica, New York: 1910, p. 791.
6. Oxford English Dictionary, Oxford: Oxford University Press, 1971, p. 1336.
7. Majno, G. *The Healing Hand.* Boston: Harvard University Press, 1975.
8. Saunders, C. *Oxford Textbook of Palliative Medicine.* Oxford: Oxford University Press, 1993.
9. Zias, J.E. "Paleopathological Evidence of Leprosy in Palestine During the Talmudic Period." *Koroth,* 9(1–2), Fall 1985.
10. Cohen, K.P. *Hospice: Prescription for Terminal Care.* Germantown, MD: Aspen Systems Corporation, 1979.
11. Casteglioni, A. *A History of Medicine.* New York: Jason Aronson, Inc., 1969.
12. Boswell, J. *The Kindness of Strangers.* New York: Pantheon Books, 1988.
13. Rosenberg, C. *The Care of Strangers.* New York: Basic Books, 1987.
14. Pernick, M.S. *A Calculus of Suffering: Pain, Professionalism, and Anesthesia in Nineteenth-Century America.* New York: Columbia University Press, 1985.
15. Encyclopedia of Bioethics. New York: Simon & Schuster, 1995.
16. Kubler-Ross, E. *On Death and Dying.* New York: Macmillan, 1969.
17. Finn Paradis, L. *The Development of Hospice in America: The Hospice Handbook.* Rockland, MD: Aspen Publications, 1985.
18. Colt, G.H. *The Enigma of Suicide.* New York: Simon & Schuster, 1991.
19. Quill, T.E. *Death and Dignity: Making Choices and Taking Charge.* New York: W.W. Norton & Co., 1993.
20. Rachels, J. *The End of Life.* Oxford: Oxford University Press, 1986.
21. Porter, R. Companion Encyclopedia of the History of Medicine. Routledge, UK, 1993, pp. 1589–1591.
22. King, H. *The History of the Management of Pain.* In Mann, R.D., ed. Park Ridge, NJ: Pantheon Publishing Group, 1988.
23. Mann, R.D. "The History of the Non-Steroidal Anti-inflammatory Agents." In Mann, R.D., ed. *The History of the Management of Pain.* Park Ridge, NJ: The Parthenon Press, 1988, pp. 77–125.
24. Nuland, S.B. *How We Die.* New York, Alfred A. Knopf, 1994.

❖ **For Further Reading**

Campbell, L. "History of the Hospice Movement." *Cancer Nursing,* 9(6):333–338, 1986.

Dicks, B. "The Contribution of Nursing to Palliative Care." *Palliative Medicine,* 4:197–203, 1990.

Dobratz, M.C. "Hospice Nursing: Present Perspectives and Future Directives." *Cancer Nursing,* 13(2):116–122, 1990.

Stoddard, S. "Hospice in the United States: An Overview." *Journal of Palliative Care,* 5(3):10–19, 1988.

# ❖ Chapter 2

# The Referral Process and Reimbursement

JUNE VERMILLON

The 1992 National Hospice Profile documented continued growth in the number of hospice programs in the United States. The number of programs rose from one in 1974 to 1,529 in 1989, 1,874 in 1991 and 1,935 in 1992. Seventy-two percent of these programs were either certified or pending certification by Medicare in 1992. Ninety-six percent of these hospices identified themselves as being nonprofit programs. This number fell to 91 percent in 1994. The corporate affiliation among hospice programs is shifting. Nineteen ninety-four data suggest a decline in independent hospices and an increase in hospices affiliated with hospitals and home health agencies. Table 2–1 outlines the changes in status from 1992 to 1994. The number of patients and families served by hospice programs has grown from 158,000 in 1985, the year of the first national hospice census, to 246,000 in 1992.[1,2]

The referral process to hospice requires awareness of the benefits and services of the hospice program. Since many health care professionals are unaware of these benefits, the hospice professionals will need to be able to explain them to others in order for all patients to have access to the hospice program. This list includes physicians, discharge planners, patients, and families. Other sources of hospice referrals include third party payers, case managers, long-term care facilities, and the community. This chapter will discuss issues vital to maintaining referrals in order to provide hospice access to the broadest group of patients. Patient and hospice profiles will be addressed as well as reimbursement issues.

TABLE 2–1  Status of Hospice Programs

|  | 1992 | 1994 |
|---|---|---|
| Independent | 49% | 40% |
| Division of hospital | 27% | 30% |
| Division of home health agency | 21% | 23% |
| Other/unidentified | 3% | 6% |

*Source:* National Hospice Organization. *Newsline,* October 1, 1994.

11

## ❖ Medicare Certification

The Health Insurance for the Aged and Disabled Act is part of the Social Security Act known as Medicare. The Department of Health and Human Services is responsible for administering the Medicare program. Most Americans who are sixty-five years of age or older qualify for this program beginning with the first day of the month in which the individual reaches age sixty-five. The same coverage is extended to individuals under age sixty-five who qualify as disabled under Title II of the Act and those with end-stage renal disease. Medicare is divided into two sections: Part A is the hospital insurance and Part B is the voluntary supplementary medical insurance. Hospice care has been a benefit under Medicare Part A since November 1, 1983.[3] Hospice programs that choose to become certified by Medicare must meet the conditions for participation and agree to follow the Medicare hospice regulations. Once a hospice is certified, Medicare conducts annual surveys to monitor continued compliance with the Medicare hospice regulations. The surveyor reviews patient charts, interdisciplinary plans of care, and other pertinent records. Home visits are made with the staff and discussions are held with members of the management team. Only Medicare certified hospices are able to offer the Medicare hospice benefit to their patients. This type of reimbursement mechanism will be described later in this chapter.

## ❖ Admission Criteria

The basic admission criteria, as formalized in the Medicare Act that funded the hospice benefit, are listed in Table 2–2. Individual hospice programs may modify the criteria to include more specific criteria. Under the Medicare hospice regulations, the hospice medical director or the physician member of the hospice interdisciplinary team and the individual's attending physician must sign a statement certifying that the individual's medical prognosis suggests a life expectancy of six months or less.[3] The attending physician, the patient, and the patient's family must be in agreement that a palliative course of treatment is the appropriate choice, rather than care aimed at prolonging life. The hospice may require a primary caregiver (family member or significant other) who will be responsible for providing or arranging for continued care when the patient is no longer able to maintain self-care activities. According to the 1992 National Hospice Profile, 45 percent of the

TABLE 2–2  Hospice Admission Criteria

| |
| --- |
| Individual is certified as being terminally ill. |
| Individual wants hospice care. |
| Physician is willing to provide medical care and consultation. |

*Source:* U.S. Department of Health and Human Services. *Medicare: Hospice Manual,* U.S. Department of Commerce National Technical Information Service, Washington, DC, 1992.

hospice programs admitted patients without primary caregivers. An additional 31 percent made this decision on a case-by-case basis.[1] Other criteria for admission may include the patient residing in the service area and the home environment being safe and conducive to the care needed. Each hospice program develops specific policies. Table 2–3 lists selected policies and compares their prevalence in 1990 to 1992. Early referral is encouraged to allow time for hospice services to be of full benefit to the patient and family.

## ❖ Profiles of Patients and Services

Of the 246,000 patients served by hospice programs in 1992, 67 percent were over the age of sixty-five, 32 percent were adults and 1 percent were children under the age of eighteen. Table 2–4 provides a profile of the patient census of an average hospice in the United States. Table 2–5 lists selected demographic information. The statistics reflect consistency with past National Hospice Organization (NHO) census data. However, cancer diagnoses have decreased from 84 percent in 1990 to 78 percent in 1992. In 1992, hospice programs indicated that 77 percent of their patients died at home, 14 percent died in acute inpatient facilities, and 9 percent in another institution. The average length of stay in the hospice program increased from fifty-nine days in 1990 to sixty-four days in 1992.[1,4]

TABLE 2–3    Policies in Hospice Programs

|                                          | 1990 | 1992 |
|------------------------------------------|------|------|
| Informed consent                         | 75%  | 98%  |
| Primary caregiver signature on admission | 74%  | N/A  |
| Primary caregiver informed consent       | 72%  | N/A  |
| Patient understanding of illness         | 59%  | N/A  |
| Do not resuscitate order                 | 39%  | 40%  |

*Sources:* National Hospice Organization. *Hospice Care in America: A Statistical Profile.* 1991; National Hospice Organization. National Hospice Profile. *Newsline,* October, 1993.

TABLE 2–4    Average Hospice Patient Census, 1990

Annual census: 130 patients

Daily home census: 25 patients

Daily inpatient census: 2 patients

Length of stay in hospice program: 59 days (1992: 64 days)

1,604 hospice patients surveyed for 1990 census.

*Sources:* National Hospice Organization. *Hospice Care in America: A Statistical Profile.* 1991; National Hospice Organization. National Hospice Profile. *Newsline,* October, 1993.

TABLE 2–5    Hospice Demographic Information

| Gender | | Racial Group | | Disease | |
|---|---|---|---|---|---|
| Men | 53% | Caucasian | 85% | Cancer | 78% |
| Women | 47% | African-American | 9% | Cardiac | 10% |
| | | Hispanic | 3% | Other | 6% |
| | | Other | 3% | Acquired Immune Deficiency Syndrome | 4% |
| | | | | Renal | 1% |
| | | | | Alzheimer's Disease | 1% |

Source: National Hospice Organization. National Hospice Profile. Newsline, October, 1993.

## ❖ Financial Reimbursement

Hospice services are financed by a variety of sources. These are listed in Table 2–6. The most common sources will be described in more detail.

### Medicare Hospice Benefit

The Medicare hospice benefit was created and shaped by hospice people and has become the major reimbursement source for hospice care in the United States. This reimbursement model has influenced the structure and delivery of hospice care. The benefit introduced the concept of managed care to hospice through the prospective per diem reimbursement structure, initiated levels of care, established minimum standards, mandated a specific mix of services to be provided, and influenced private insurance plans to cover hospice care.

The Medicare hospice benefit was established in 1983 for terminally ill patients. The patient waives Medicare Part A to elect the Medicare hospice benefit for all care related to the terminal illness. Hospice then becomes totally responsible for the determination and care of that patient's medical and supportive care needs related to the terminal illness. Standard Medicare remains in effect to cover all care not related to the terminal illness. There is no limit on the number of days a patient may remain in the hospice program under Medicare. The Medicare hospice benefit is divided into four periods. The first and second periods are ninety days each. The third period is thirty days and the fourth period is indefinite, but if the patient revokes (i.e., chooses to leave during this later period), the hospice program can no longer be reimbursed by Medicare. The patient is monitored closely at the end of each period for appropriateness for hospice care in regard to the six-month life expectancy.[3] Hospice patients may enter and remain in the program throughout the course of their illness or may choose to leave the program

TABLE 2–6   Reimbursement Sources

|                                        | 1990 | 1993 |
|----------------------------------------|------|------|
| Medicare                               | 65%  | 68%  |
| Private health insurance               | 22%  | 13%  |
| Other (includes indigent and self pay) | 9%   | 12%  |
| Medicaid hospice benefit               | 4%   | 7%   |

*Sources:* National Hospice Organization 1990 Census; National Hospice Organization 1993 Census.

after a period of time and return later. These decisions are made within the context of discussions between the interdisciplinary team, the patient, and the family. Unlike standard Medicare, the Medicare hospice benefit has no requirement that a patient must be homebound. In fact, hospice workers support the patient and family by encouraging activities outside the home that enhance their quality of life. This may be in a shopping trip or a visit to family or friends. Children in the hospice program often continue to attend school. The Medicare hospice benefit provides payment for hospice beneficiaries, on a per diem basis according to the level of care provided. In 1990, approximately 53 percent of hospice patients were enrolled on the benefit.[3,4] Medicare regulations include a 5 percent co-pay to be collected from the patient on inpatient respite days and pharmaceuticals.[3] Each hospice determines whether or not this will be collected. The NHO and the Hospice Association of America (HAA) have been successful in obtaining rate increases for each type of care setting. The annual rate increases are tied to the "hospital market basket" index. The Medicare hospice benefit includes four levels of care: routine home care, continuous home care, general inpatient care, and inpatient respite care. The care provided in each setting will be described in more detail in Chapter 6.

The routine home care per diem rate is designed to cover the cost of all hospice visits, supplies, medications, and services. The Medicare conditions of participation define a distinctive cluster of services that the hospice must provide regardless of the care setting. These are listed in Table 2–7. Other treatments and services are covered according to the individual plan of care. They may include intravenous therapy, blood transfusions, and palliative radiation therapy. Hospices often require that specific treatments be preauthorized by the interdisciplinary team. The hospice nurse is usually the team member who is responsible for coordinating medications, supplies, equipment, and treatments.

The coverage under the continuous home care rate is intended to provide a combination of skilled nursing (RNs) and personal care (home health aides) in the home during periods of "medical crisis." A period of crisis is defined as a time when the patient requires continuous care to achieve palliation or management of acute medical symptoms.

TABLE 2–7    Medicare Required Hospice Services

Interdisciplinary team

Medicines and biologicals

Laboratory services

X-ray and radiation therapy

Emergency services

Ambulance and transport services

Bereavement support

*Source:* U.S. Department of Health and Human Services. *Medicare: Hospice Manual*, U.S. Department of Commerce National Technical Information Service, Washington, DC, 1992.

Inpatient general days are utilized for the home-care patient whose pain or symptoms cannot be controlled at home. The average length of stay for these patients is five to seven days. Hospices carefully monitor inpatient admissions, which are intended under the Medicare benefit to be infrequent and short term. Medicare regulations require that no more than 20 percent of total aggregate patient days be inpatient general days.[3]

Inpatient respite services are available to provide short-term (up to five days) relief for the caregiver. Inpatient respite stays can be provided in a hospital on a dedicated hospice unit or other division or in a long-term care facility through a contractual agreement. Respite can also be provided in a hospice facility.

The Medicare hospice regulations also established qualifications for how hospice care is provided. The conditions are listed in Table 2–8. The patient or representative may revoke the Medicare hospice benefit at any time during the benefit period. The patient loses hospice coverage for the remainder of the benefit period, but may re-elect hospice coverage at any time for those periods that he or she is still eligible to receive. At the time of revocation, the patient resumes coverage under standard Medicare.[3]

## Medicaid Hospice Benefit

In 1986, legislation was passed allowing the states to develop coverage for hospice programs. According to the 1990 National Hospice Census, 4 percent of the patients served by certified hospices listed Medicaid as the source of reimbursement.[4] Thirty-six states have implemented the Medicaid hospice benefit, which is patterned after the Medicare hospice benefit in services and reimbursement. The Medicaid hospice benefit does not include co-payment for inpatient respite stays or pharmaceuticals. For this reason Medicaid per diem payments are slightly higher than Medicare payments on routine day and inpatient respite day levels of care. Another area in which Medicaid differs primarily is in offering services to Medicaid qualified nursing home residents. The hospice receives reimbursement for pro-

Table 2–8    Medicare Requirements for Hospice Care

Continuity of care

Informed consent

Continuation of care regardless of ability to pay

Access to all levels of hospice care

Patient rights

*Source:* U.S. Department of Health and Human Services. *Medicare: Hospice Manual,* U.S. Department of Commerce National Technical Information Service, Washington, DC, 1992.

viding hospice Medicaid services in addition to "room and board" funds to pay for basic nursing home housing for the patient. The hospice then becomes the financial guarantor for the individual's nursing home expenses. Hospices may see a change in Medicaid reimbursement as some states move to privatize state-funded health care.

## Private Insurance

Private insurers, Health Maintenance Organizations (HMOs) and Preferred Provider Organizations (PPOs) are presently exploring hospice benefits for their patients and seeking programs experienced in managing care and costs. Coverage of hospice services under private insurance plans varies by individual policy. If they offer a hospice benefit, the majority of private insurance companies provides reimbursement per visit and usually covers nursing, social service, and home health aide visits. With managed care and case managers, hospices are seeing increased negotiations for comprehensive per diem reimbursement.

## Veterans Health Administration

On January 6, 1992, the Veterans Health Administration (VHA) called on the nation's 172 VA Medical Centers (VAMC) to begin offering hospice care to their terminally ill patients.[5] The VA plan was to provide access to an organized and coordinated program of hospice care at every medical center by the end of the 1993 fiscal year. VA medical facilities could provide hospice care by establishing their own programs or by working with existing community-based hospices. Special components of the VHA directive described a hospice consultation team (HCT), inpatient hospice care for patients without caregivers, and a designated inpatient unit with home care capability. It is left to each VAMC to decide the complexity of hospice services appropriate to that particular institution. A minimal requirement is to have an HCT at each VAMC. The HCT is to consult, coordinate, and refer veterans for hospice services. The home care component of the directive listed referral of eligible veterans to community-based hospices under Medicare or

Medicaid eligibility, purchase of community-based hospice care for veterans eligible for fee-basis care, or referral to hospital-based home care (HBHC) at medical centers where they can provide care to those with a terminal illness. Since September 1993, some VAMC and community-based hospices have created successful linkages to provide hospice home care to eligible veterans who remain at home for hospice care.[6] Working with VAMC to provide home care hospice services to veterans creates opportunities and challenges. The opportunities are to serve a new group of hospice beneficiaries and the challenges are to negotiate with the VAMC on the special situations that arise with specific patients.

## Acceptance Regardless of Ability to Pay

NHO has suggested that palliative care should be available to all terminally ill patients regardless of their ability to pay for these services.[7] Hospices are creative in developing resources to fund their services. Most hospice programs provide services based on need rather than ability to pay. Patients who do not have medical insurance may be billed according to a sliding fee scale. Costs incurred by the hospice program, as well as the difference between cost of services and payment provided by insurance, are offset by philanthropic dollars. These monies are established through memorial contributions, donations from individuals, corporations, community service groups, and fund-raising projects within the community.

### Community Funding

Philanthropic contributions from a variety of sources continue to provide important support for hospice programs. United Way provides approximately 14 percent of the philanthropic support monies for hospice programs across the country.[1]

Memorial donations are another major source of support for hospice programs, providing 26 percent of philanthropic dollars.[1] Families frequently list hospice as the charity of choice for contributions after the death of the patient. The value of the hospice program is often validated with cards and letters.

Specific campaigns, including capital campaigns, provide 26 percent of philanthropic dollars to hospice programs. Fund raising activities also provide funds; the activities vary among hospice programs and demonstrate the creativity of those involved in this work.

### ❖ Summary

Hospice care is provided to terminally ill individuals and their families by nearly 2,000 hospice programs in the United States. The majority of patients have cancer, although this number is decreasing as more patients enter hospice programs with other life-threatening illnesses. Anyone may refer an individual to a hospice program by simply calling a local hospice. Hospice care is based on need rather than the ability to pay. However, Medicare, Medicaid, some private insurance companies, and philanthropic money provide reimbursement for hospice care.

## ❖ References

1. National Hospice Organization. National Hospice Profile. *Newsline,* October, 1993.
2. National Hospice Organization. *Newsline,* October 1, 1994.
3. *Medicare: Hospice Manual,* U.S. Department of Health and Human Services. U.S. Department of Commerce National Technical Information Service, Washington, DC, 1992.
4. National Hospice Organization. *Hospice Care in America: A Statistical Profile.* 1991.
5. Veterans Health Administration Directive 10-92-001. Department of Veterans Affairs. Plans for Hospice Care of the Terminally Ill Veteran. January 6, 1992.
6. Veterans Health Administration Directive 10-92-091. Department of Veterans Affairs. Policy on Implementation of Hospice Programs. September 9, 1992.
7. *Standards of a Hospice Program of Care.* National Hospice Organization. Arlington, VA: 1993.

# ❖ Chapter 3
# The Interdisciplinary Team

Jeanne M. Martinez

Over the past twenty years, hospital-based inpatient care has adopted interdisciplinary care as a preferred model for addressing patients' complex health care needs. This concept followed "consumerism" and the "women's movement," both originating in the 1960s when consumers identified the need to become more active and assertive in many arenas. This activism impacted health care with a change from a paternalistic view of the physician-patient relationship to one where the patient was considered a partner and thus a member of the team in prevention, treatment, and healing. This concept also changed the relationship among physicians, nurses and other health care providers. Each discipline has expertise to contribute to the care of the patient and family. The goal of the interdisciplinary team is to work with patients to identify their specific needs and health goals within a holistic framework. Each member contributes from their unique areas of practice rather than focusing on treatment of disease entities or resolution of physical symptoms in isolation. The interdisciplinary team concept varies widely in practice in acute medicine. However, hospice care has been purposely designed to require the initial consultation and necessary follow-up care of an interdisciplinary team.[1]

## ❖ Interview Process

A variety of issues should be discussed during the initial interview of prospective candidates regardless of their potential roles in hospice. It is important to determine whether they have had a personal loss within the past year. These individuals may concentrate on their own personal needs rather than on the needs of the patient and their family. Therefore, it is important to discuss the personal loss at the time of interview. Much of the information gathered from the potential candidate in the initial interview can become part of the screening process. Discussing personal interests, reasons for applying for a particular position, communication style, support system, team concept, and ability to work with dying patients is essential for determining whether the person is appropriate for hospice work and how he or she might best serve as a team member. The interview process should also focus on how the candidate receives support, copes, and relieves stress. This discussion is very important because, in order to provide quality care for the dying, the hospice workers must be able to care for themselves.

Discussing conflict resolution and the team approach in the initial interview may assist in the selection of team members who will handle conflict in a constructive, positive manner with direct communication and who will be interactive and cooperative team members. Direct communication and conflict resolution assists in appropriate communication and creates effectiveness when working within the team structure. A close bond is often created between the hospice team members and the patients and their families. Therefore, the ability to set professional limits is extremely important and should be explored. Failure to set limits is detrimental to the team approach, to the patient and family, and to the team members. Patients and their families may ask the home health aide or volunteer to do things that may be more personal in nature. Setting limits allows for open communication and assists in providing a comprehensive approach to hospice care.

## ❖ Members of the Team

Hospice in the United States began largely as a self-described consumer movement. Therefore, it is no surprise that the patient and family are identified in hospice standards as the center of the team. The patient's attending physician is also a member of the team. Medicare hospice regulations define the following as core services: physician services, nursing services, medical social services, and counseling services. These services must be directly provided by hospice employees; that is, the care cannot be provided by contract arrangement except in times of peak patient loads or under extraordinary circumstances. The Medicare hospice regulations further specify the composition and role of the interdisciplinary team. The team must be composed of a doctor of medicine or osteopathy, a registered nurse, a social worker, and a pastoral or other counselor. Each team is facilitated by a patient care coordinator or team leader. The responsibilities of the interdisciplinary team are outlined in Table 3–1. If the hospice program has more than one interdisciplinary team, it must designate those individuals responsible for establishing the policies that govern the provision of hospice care and services. Hospice must make nursing services, physician services and medications, and biologicals routinely available on a twenty-four-hour basis. Other covered services must also be available on a twenty-four-hour basis to the extent necessary to meet the specific needs of the individuals served in the hospice program. In addition, the

TABLE 3–1    Responsibilities of the Interdisciplinary Hospice Team

Participate in the establishment of the plan of care

Provide or supervise hospice care and services

Review and update the plan of care

Establish policies governing hospice care and services

*Source: Medicare: Hospice Manual.* U.S. Department of Health and Human Services. U.S. Department of Commerce National Technical Information Service, Washington, DC, 1992.

following services must be made available to patients as needed, although they may be provided on a contract basis: occupational therapy, physical therapy, speech therapy, dietary consultation, homemakers, and home health aides.[1]

Some hospices offer additional services that are not outlined in the Medicare hospice regulations. These include, but are not limited to, music therapy, art therapy, massage therapy, and financial counseling. Medical specialists such as neurosurgeons, anesthesiologists, and psychiatrists may also be included as consultants for specific problems. Volunteers are considered hospice employees. They must provide direct patient care or administrative support of patient care activities such as clerical work in the hospice office. The services provided for each patient are based on the interdisciplinary care plan. Therefore, the team members are determined by each patient's needs at any given point in time. The patient may only need the services provided by the core team members when they enter the hospice program. A home health aide may be needed later to assist with bathing and a music therapist to guide and teach relaxation techniques.

## Hospice Medical Director

At a minimum each hospice must have a physician designated as the medical director. This physician has both administrative and clinical responsibilities. Administratively, the medical director reviews hospice policies and participates in quality assurance studies. Under Medicare regulations, the medical director is responsible for determining the medical eligibility of patients for hospice care, and certifying (initially in collaboration with one other physician) that the patient is terminally ill. The medical director must be consulted on each patient's initial plan of care and is responsible for recertifying patients for subsequent benefit periods to continue their hospice benefits under Medicare. The medical director must also be available to provide primary care to the patient if the patient's physician is unable to carry out this role. Beyond these required functions, the effective medical director must have expertise in pain and symptom management, a strong knowledge base in a primary field of medicine, comfort with difficult emotional issues, and the ability to communicate compassion and empathy. Good communication skills are also required to provide consultation and support to referring physicians and foster cohesive collaboration within the hospice team.

## Nurse

Nurse coordination drives most patient services and care. The nurse must continually evaluate the need for medical supplies, durable medical equipment, therapy, and counseling. The nurse needs good physical assessment skills and a working knowledge of pain and symptom management appropriate to palliative care. This must include the emotional and spiritual dimensions of patient comfort, and a focus on quality of life *as defined by the patient*.

## Medical Social Worker

Although a medical social worker is a required member of the team, the role of the social worker in hospice practice may vary widely. At a minimum, the social worker must review each patient's care plan upon admission to the hospice program and provide an initial psychosocial assessment of the patient and family. This assessment contributes to the identified patient and family problem list, usually focusing on emotional, legal, financial, and, at times, spiritual needs. These identified issues then determine the extent of the social worker's involvement with the patient and family. The psychosocial assessment also provides the beginning of the bereavement assessment. Depending on the structure of the individual hospice program, the social worker may have a major role in providing spiritual care, support to the family at the time of death, and grief counseling—particularly for those individuals assessed as "high-risk" for complicated bereavement. Larger programs employ spiritual care coordinators to facilitate this care by specially trained volunteers. Many programs also employ health care professionals from a variety of disciplines as bereavement counselors or coordinators. These roles are discussed in more detail in Chapter 4.

## Counselor

This role is defined by Medicare and other hospice regulatory bodies as a pastoral or other counselor. This position is often occupied by a person who represents the clergy and is perhaps the least defined of the core team members. In practice, this team member is expected to have expertise in counseling patients and family members on grief and loss issues, as well as addressing spiritual concerns. This individual is also responsible for identifying and communicating with community clergy to best meet individual patient needs. In some programs, the counselor may have the additional responsibility of providing support to hospice staff and volunteers. The spiritual care coordinator usually provides or uses appropriate resources to meet the religious and spiritual needs of the patient.

## Volunteers

Hospice is the only Medicare program that mandates volunteer care.[1] Although volunteers may be health care professionals, they most often are lay people from every conceivable walk of life. Volunteers provide a multitude of services within hospice programs, ranging from hands-on caregiving to working in the hospice office and assisting with fund-raising and public relations activities. All these functions are valuable to hospice. However, the Medicare mandate specifically refers to hands-on care, which must constitute a minimum of 5 percent of total hospice staff hours. Medicare and most state licensing regulations also specify which aspects of volunteer training the hospice program is required to provide before utilizing individuals as volunteers. Volunteers may function best for hospice in continually providing a lay perspective for the professional caregivers on the team. Most hospices employ a volunteer coordinator to orchestrate the volunteers in a variety of roles.

## ❖ Staff Characteristics

Regardless of discipline, all hospice practitioners and volunteers should be screened and selected by similar criteria beyond their individual professional expertise. It is essential to look for individuals who balance their lives on a number of levels. For example, interest in working with patients with life-threatening illnesses is obviously required. However, an extremely intense or obsessive interest is a red flag that a candidate may be inappropriate for hospice work. Hospice caregivers must be empathetic. They should be hard-working but pursue leisure activities outside of work. Home hospice care requires a unique blend of someone comfortable with working independently, and at times in isolation, yet who can participate enthusiastically as part of a team. Professional turf issues have no place in hospice care, as high-functioning hospice teams often require members to blur their roles because many responsibilities overlap. Professionals and volunteers who have worked through their own past grief experience may have much to offer others who are grieving; however, sometimes those with unresolved grief will seek out hospice work before they are ready. A loss inventory should be part of every hospice screening tool for staff and volunteers. Other motivations for hospice work should also be investigated. As with prospective employees, personal and business references should be obtained on all volunteer candidates prior to acceptance into hospice volunteer training. Many hospice programs utilize communication exercises during volunteer training to further evaluate each candidate's appropriateness and motivation for volunteering. All hospice workers need to be good communicators and especially good listeners. All staff need to be trained and evaluated in this area. Staff and volunteers should be made aware of how necessary good communication is for effective functioning of the team. Effective team members are prepared and willing to be supportive of their colleagues as needed. Some hopice programs offer staff support groups. This concept will be described in more detail in Chapter 13. It cannot be overemphasized to candidates in the interview process that hospice work is often inherently difficult and emotionally draining. Individuals should be taught the responsibility of asking for assistance for themselves when needed, whether that assistance is technical or emotional. Hospice personnel need to help each other identify potential or actual emotional issues that may affect individual or group functioning or patient care. Each individual needs to develop his or her own coping strategies. Above all, hospice programs should communicate the value of taking care of oneself as a fundamental ingredient for providing excellent hospice care.

### ❖ The Team in Action

For those who care for individuals in their homes, the only time the entire team can physically work together is at team conferences. As one mechanism for assuring interdisciplinary care, Medicare hospice regulations[1] require that a formal team conference be conducted to review each patient every two weeks. For most programs, patient acuity and short-term patient stays make weekly team conferences a necessity. Medicare also requires written evidence of care-planning at these team meetings. Meeting minutes are not sufficient to meet this written requirement. Each involved team member must document updates on a care plan summary form for each patient reviewed. Aside from meeting regulatory requirements, the size of the program often dictates the formality, content, and length of team conference. Some programs incorporate a strict format for patient review. Others allow an informal format, recognizing staff members' need to tell their story, support one another, and enjoy the social aspects of team conferences. Team conferences can also serve as mini-inservices, discussing issues such as pain and symptom management and spiritual distress. When reviewing patients who require particularly complex problem solving and interventions, team conferences can model the best of interdisciplinary care. In addition, team conferences may be the ideal or only time that most hospice staff members can come together to hear a bereavement report, if this is incorporated into team conference. Often, the most positive feedback from families comes after the patient's death during bereavement follow-up visits or telephone calls. Staff may use this feedback as a mechanism to evaluate their patient care. It may also give individual staff members a different perspective in situations where they felt they were ineffective by actually hearing in the bereavement period how supported family members felt. Each program needs to develop its own structure and philosophy about team conference. The conference's structure and purpose then needs to be clarified for the staff. Most interdisciplinary care occurs outside of the formal team conference; team members must be able to trust each other to provide appropriate assessment and timely intervention. When this does not happen, team members need to confront these issues with each other, and when necessary, with supervisory staff. When conflicts are ignored, the team process will be impaired. An example of a structure for team conference is outlined in Table 3–2.

### ❖ Family Conferences

Hospice care commonly begins with a family conference. The patient identifies the important friends and family members who will be involved in caretaking and decision making. Initiating hospice care involves discussion of difficult emotional issues and decisions. It is common for patients and family members to try to protect each other from emotionally

TABLE 3–2   A Structure for a Hospice Team Conference

| Bereavement Report | Current Patient Report | New Patients |
|---|---|---|
| Bereavement coordinator reports on family follow-up. Primary or on-call nurse reports on deaths that have occurred since the last team conference. | Patient care coordinator facilitates the team conference. Primary nurse begins with patient's name, age, diagnosis, and current problems, then asks, "Who else has seen the patient this week?" Team members add their comments, including identification of additional problems and interventions. Team members may ask questions or give input. | Patients who are new to the program since the last team conference are presented by the assessment nurse, patient care coordinator, or primary nurse. |

painful information. Initial contact with the patient and family together helps identify communication and coping styles, as well as current areas of conflict among family members. A family conference is most helpful in facilitating communication between all persons involved in the care of the individual. It is most helpful in beginning to break down communication barriers when they exist. The components of a family conference are listed in Table 3–3. The initial conference should include written materials about the program's services, including specifics about the Medicare or other insurance benefits available to a particular patient. Generally, consent forms are also reviewed at this time. Some programs utilize a primary caregiver consent form that spells out this person's responsibilities in working with the hospice team in the care of the patient. Subsequent family conferences generally occur either because there are problems in the care of the patient at home, or because many family members are involved, requiring communication to be focused. These conferences must be carefully arranged, so that all appropriate parties can attend. To emphasize the concept of team care, it is most helpful to have more than one hospice team member attend a family conference. Ideally this should be the patient's physician, the primary hospice nurse, and an involved social worker or hospice counselor. The specific team members are determined by the focus of the conference. When family conferences are necessary after the initial meeting, the topics can range from bathing to exhaustion of the caregivers. Family conferences are an effective means of problem-solving, redirecting care, and clarifying issues concerning barriers to patient care.

TABLE 3–3    Components of Family Conference

Clarification that both patient and family understand the terminal nature of the illness

Current concerns of the patient and each family member

Patient's and family members' expectations of the hospice program

Specific services the hospice can provide

Identifying the patient's and family members' goals for care and how the hospice can help to meet them

Expectations the hospice program has of the patient and family

## ❖ Office Space and Equipment

Space needs will be determined by the size and general scope of the program. Programs may develop a community bereavement or education focus. Some programs decide to provide their own durable medical equipment (DME), effectively becoming a DME vendor. The small volunteer program common in the early days of hospice is rare. Most current programs are competitive and run with the efficiency common in the world of business. Computerized data management is a necessity for all but the very smallest of programs. Programs should plan for the computerization of clinical records because this technology is fast becoming available. Lap-top computers and cellular phones are optional but strongly recommended for home care staff. Independent programs must be able to store medical records and some medical supplies. Nursing bags stocked according to regulations should be provided. An adequately sized conference room and the usual office paraphernalia are necessities. Finally, private space should be provided for counseling patients and families and other work that requires a closed door.

## ❖ Summary

Hospice care has been designed to provide holistic care by an interdisciplinary health care team that includes lay volunteers and professional caregivers. The patient, family members, and the patient's attending physician are also part of this team. Hospice staff and volunteers must balance the ability to work independently with the responsibility of being part of the team. In addition to the office space and supplies required by most home care agencies, adequate conference room space for team meetings and private counseling space are necessary for hospice care. New technology such as computerized medical records and cellular phones can further enhance effective hospice work in the community. It is imperative for hospice programs to screen, select, and prepare staff for the emotional and technical aspects of care. Volunteers also require careful screening and training for the rewarding and intensely emotional work of caring for the dying and their families. Interdependence and collaboration are the cornerstones to a strong interdisciplinary team. As the team works together by learning from one another and supporting and encouraging each other, a sense of competence and self-confidence will develop to provide a creative team and individual growth.[2]

## ❖ References

1. *Medicare: Hospice Manual.* U.S. Department of Health and Human Services. U.S. Department of Commerce National Technical Information Service, Washington, DC, 1992.
2. Dunlop, R.J., and Hockley, J.M. *Terminal Care Support Teams.* Oxford: Oxford University Press, 1990.

# ❖ Chapter 4
# The Core Team

GARY A. JOHANSON
INES V. JOHANSON

As we attempt to apply the compassion and science of palliative care to the relief of suffering in dying patients, it is helpful to reflect upon Cassell's[1] observation that suffering is a truly complex dimension that occurs when an impending future destruction of any portion of the person is perceived. The dimensions of personhood he describes include physical, emotional, past, future, transcendent, and others. No one person begins to have the time, interest, or experience to be able to address all the potential sources of suffering. Thus, the team approach to palliative and hospice care has emerged.

The size of an interdisciplinary hospice team varies depending upon the resources and philosophy of the hospice program, as well as the needs of the patients and their families. Medicare formalized the hospice team by mandating certain core members in their hospice regulations.[2] This core group is composed of a physician, registered nurse, social worker, and pastoral or other counselor. A hospice may include as many individuals as it chooses in order to meet the needs of the patients and their families. Not only do members of this team have differing skills and insights, but as a consequence of who they are, they provide a spectrum of personalities with whom patients can hope to connect with their myriads of problems, challenges, and concerns.

## ❖ Physician

Although physical and psychosocial symptoms must be assessed and treated simultaneously, the relief of physical symptoms provides opportunities for patients to explore areas of emotional, social, and spiritual suffering more fully. It is here that the physician serves as one of the key members of the interdisciplinary team. The most common roles for a physician include hospice medical director, attending physician, and team physician. In most hospice programs, the attending and team physician are members of the core team. The physician is trained and experienced to assess the interactions between the various pathophysiologic problems (e.g., cancer of the lung, chronic obstructive lung disease, and the use of morphine). With this assessment, the team can assist the patient in choosing among the treatment options. The physician is often most knowledgeable in regard to potentially reversible situations (e.g., hypercalcemia as a cause of coma).

## Medical Director

The role of the medical director varies greatly depending on the degree and scope to which physicians and other interdisciplinary team members collaborate. Factors contributing to this wide variability are listed in Table 4–1. The primary role of the medical director is to provide guidance, support, and medical direction in the development of interdisciplinary care plans and the ongoing care of patients. The medical director should be available to nurses for collaboration on patient related problems twenty-four hours a day. Depending on the culture of the community, the medical director may consult informally with community physicians on occasional patient palliative care needs, or may become more formally involved with the direct care of many terminally ill patients. When an inpatient unit is a part of the program, direct patient care and supervision will take on an even larger portion of a physician's responsibilities. The attending physician or the medical director will follow the patient in the unit. Guidance on clinical issues goes well beyond symptom relief issues, often delving deeply into ethical issues and fundamental decisions on pathways of treatment. The medical director may assist in the formulation and presentation of educational programs to the general and professional communities. This individual may also participate in hospice workshops and inservices for staff and volunteers. The hospice medical director may also serve as a professional and community liaison.

As hospice and palliative care are integrated more and more into mainstream medicine, the hospice physician plays a paramount role in promoting and facilitating healthy dialogue between palliative care teams and the physician community at large. The medical director is in a key position to represent hospice services to the medical community. This is often done through one-to-one dialogue. Individuals on either side of the treat-to-cure and treat-for-comfort spectrum of care often need tactful and skillful assistance in understanding each other's point of view and how it translates best into appropriae patient care. The literature is calling more and more for a tighter integration of palliative medicine into the medical system and cancer centers.[3,4] The World Health Organization suggests that many aspects of palliative care may be applied in conjunction with anticancer treatment earlier

TABLE 4–1  Factors Affecting the Role of the Medical Director

Philosophy of the Board of Directors and management

Perceived value of physician involvement

Budgetary considerations

Availability of other physicians with the skills, interest, and time to devote to the team

The comfort level of the interdisciplinary team members in working with physicians in the course of the illness.[5] It is important to liaison well with the general community so that the potential negative death connotations of hospice can be optimally dispelled. The medical director also plays a role in program development, working with the managing leadership of a hospice program in the development of policies and procedures involving all the clinical aspects of the program. Many of the policies are required by certifying bodies or agencies and require physician attention on an ongoing basis. The Medicare hospice certification process is one example. Utilization review and quality assurance activities are important aspects of a medical director's duties as well as involvement in clinical research.

The medical director also can be an important source of support to the members of the interdisciplinary team and to patients and their families. He or she may provide reassurance that what is being done is right for that patient. This is often done through collaboration with the hospice team. The qualifications of the medical director are listed in Table 4–2, the responsibilities in Table 4–3.

TABLE 4–2    Qualifications of a Hospice Medical Director

Current license in the state of practice

Knowledge and diagnostic skills in a primary care medical discipline

Additional training in oncology, pharmacology, and palliative medicine

Understanding of family counseling and psychological responses to grief and loss

Experience in working with terminally ill patients

Knowledge of local medical community

Ability to communicate effectively with medical peers

Willingness to make home visits

Ability to be supportive and empathize with patients, families, and staff

Ability to work diplomatically with a wide range of personalities and situations

Ability to work within and contribute to an interdisciplinary team

Ability to cope with stress and ambiguity

TABLE 4–3    Responsibilities of the Medical Director

Medical consultation

Education

Community and professional liaison

Program development

Support and guidance

## Hospice Team Physician

One or more team physicians, possessing special interest and experience in palliative medicine, may be available to an interdisciplinary team and attending physician. He or she can assist the medical director with clinical issues or administrative duties. Some large hospice programs employ physicians for this role.

## Attending Physician

The patient's primary physician remains an integral part of the patient's care team and is designated as the patient's attending physician.[6] The physician can bring information regarding the patient's medical history and its impact on the individual's life to the team. He or she may also be a stable and trusted resource to the patient and family, a relationship which often only develops over time. The attending physician collaborates primarily with the patient's hospice nurse and may also interact with the hospice team physician or medical director on complex symptom management or ethics and philosophy of care issues.

## ❖ Registered Nurse

Many of the qualities which attract people to nursing are also the qualities so finely suited to the practice of hospice nursing. Nursing practice has always brought together multiple components of health care delivery in its approach to patient care. These include clinical issues, nurturing, spiritual concerns, teaching, and patient advocacy. All of these are part of the continuum of nursing practice. Hospice offers nurses the opportunity as well as the responsibility to engage in the many issues which face patients and their families. This becomes particularly important because advanced diseases can alter lifestyles and self image. It is here that the full spectrum of nursing practice comes into play by going beyond physical assessment and delivery of prescribed treatment to include the psychological aspects of disease and the impact which such stressors impart on overall function.[7] Hospice nursing requires special knowledge, training, and skills. Dobratz describes four categories which define and describe the hospice nurse.[8] They are listed in Table 4-4. It is in the development of the interdisciplinary plan of care where the nurse assists the patient and family members to identify their needs. The plan of care should assist a patient and family with optimum adaptation to illness as well as promotion of comfort and independence. The hospice nurse is in an ideal position to affect coping mechanisms which encompass the person's need for adequate information concerning their disease and symptoms and retention of as much control as possible over their environment and themselves.[9] Physical symptoms must be accurately assessed and interventions must be initiated quickly and proceed in logical sequence. The nurse must have the knowledge and skill to modify the plan of care as the disease progresses. The experienced hospice nurse is

TABLE 4–4   Attributes of a Hospice Nurse

Capacity to manage physical, psychological, social, and spiritual problems of dying patients and their families

Ability to coordinate the extended and expanded components of hospice services

Acquisition of the counseling, managing, instructing, caring and communicating skills/knowledge

Ability to balance the nurse's self-care needs with the complexities and intensities of repeated encounters with death

Source: Dobratz, M.C. "Hospice Nursing: Present Perspectives and Future Directives." *Cancer Nursing*, 13(2):116–122, 1990.

able to communicate the needs of the patient and family to the members of the interdisciplinary team. In hospice, nurses gain experience essential to maximize their ability to provide holistic care.

During the last few years, there has been a move toward the development of a certification process for hospice nurses in the United States.[10,11] The process was initiated by the Hospice Nurses Association (HNA) in 1990 with the support of other hospice nursing organizations across the country, including the Academy of Hospice Nurses and the Michigan Hospice Nurses Association. The examination was developed by the National Board for Certification of Hospice Nurses (NBCHN). The examination was offered for the first time in March 1994. Four hundred eighty-two hospice nurses successfully passed the examination, thereby earning the credentials CRNH (Certified Registered Nurse Hospice).

## Primary Care Nurse

Most hospices hire registered nurses as the primary care nurse for a specific number of patients. They are responsible for the nursing care of those patients as well as the supervision of the home health aides working with the patient. These nurses may have several roles including assessment and on-call, as well as administrative duties.

## Assessment Nurse

Some of the larger hospice programs hire registered nurses specifically to make the first home visit to admit the patient into the hospice program. This visit may include a description of the program followed by expectations of the patient and family. It is important to discuss hospice philosophy and agree to the expectations of the family in regard to what the hospice program can provide. The assessment nurse may also complete a medical history, physical examination, and a brief psychosocial assessment. The goal of the visit is to begin to develop a holistic picture of the patient and family and begin the interdisciplinary plan of care. In some cases, the social worker may make a joint visit with the assessment nurse.

## On-Call Nurse

The on-call nurse responds to the needs of hospice patients and their families either by telephone or home visits during off hours. This role meets the requirement for twenty-four hour availability of nursing services outlined in the Medicare hospice regulations.[2] The on-call nurse provides assistance consistent with the plan of care. He or she visits the patient in cases of emergency or death, and is available for any other contingencies.

The structure of the on-call system is defined by the hospice program. In some programs the primary care nurses rotate through the on-call position. In others the on-call position is separate and one or more nurses are hired for this role. Large hospices often employ nurses to triage telephone calls and other nurses to make home visits. In the last case, home health aides and social workers may also make home visits as decided by the triage nurse.

Nurses may also work in the referral office or hold positions in management, human resources, public relations, or education. The qualifications of a hospice nurse are outlined in Table 4–5.

## ❖ Social Worker

The philosophy of social work encompasses the values and principles embodied in hospice. The social worker is responsible for identification of family and community systems and referral to appropriate community resources. The social worker may also counsel the patient and family on financial issues, advance directives, or psychosocial issues. Additionally, he or she may provide support and direction to team members faced with interfamily or interteam conflict. The social worker is expected to prepare a com-

---

TABLE 4–5    Qualifications of a Hospice Nurse

Current licensure in the state of practice

Minimum of one year of clinical practice in nursing. Oncology, psychiatry, and home care experience are preferred

Knowledge of pathophysiology and disease progression

Understanding of pain and symptom management

Excellent assessment and communication skills

Ability to work within and contribute to an interdisciplinary team

Ability to assist the patient and family in coping with emotional stress

Understanding of and aptitude for organization and communication with patient, family, and team members

Ability to work within the patient and family's belief system and tolerance for individual values and lifestyles

---

prehensive psychosocial assessment and organize a strategy to approach the problems which may include the appropriateness of caring for the patient at home. The qualifications of a social worker are listed in Table 4–6. It is important to note that qualifications vary depending on licensure and certification requirements specific to a particular state. Some states require certification, others require licensure.

## ❖ Counselor

The Medicare hospice regulations require a counselor to be a member of the interdisciplinary team.[2] Usually this role is occupied by a chaplain or spiritual counselor. However, social workers, nurses, and physicians may also counsel patients and family members. In some hospices, one of these individuals might have special qualifications in bereavement counseling.

### Chaplain

The chaplain may be the spiritual advisor for patients, families, and the interdisciplinary team. This individual must be a skilled listener and meet patients where they are in their own spiritual belief system. The chaplain should be able to elicit and respond to questions of meaning, guilt, disappointment, loss, the mystery of life, and fears about the future. He or she must be concerned with the fundamental emotional and activating principles of a person. These may include an individual's deepest relationships with themselves, others, and perhaps a higher being. A chaplain may also serve as a resource for patients by knowing which religious clergy person will best serve the person's needs. A chaplain may assist the interdisciplinary team to deal with issues of meaning as they care for patients and their families. Education encompassing spiritual issues is part of the hospice chaplaincy. As a nonmedical person, a chaplain brings an important community/consumer perspective to the interdisciplinary team.[12] The qualifications of a hospice chaplain are listed in Table 4–7.

TABLE 4–6  Qualifications of a Social Worker

| |
| --- |
| Bachelor's degree from an accredited school of social work |
| Masters of Social Work or a Masters of Science/Arts in Marriage and Family Counseling (recommendations of NHO) |
| A minimum of one to three years supervised experience in the health care field |
| Ability to work within and contribute to an interdisciplinary team |
| Understanding and compassion toward patients and families |
| Knowledge of community resources available to patients and their families |

TABLE 4–7   Qualifications of a Chaplain

---

Graduate of accredited seminary or school of theology, or appropriate certification in clinical pastoral education

Mature in own belief system; ability to be open and flexible, ecumenical but not evangelistic in ministry

Experience working with patients and families facing life threatening illness

Knowledge of spiritual effects of terminal illness, grief, and loss

Ability to respond compassionately and sensitively to patient and family members

Ability to work within and contribute to an interdisciplinary team

---

## Bereavement Counselor

Educational and training programs are available to bereavement counselors. Specifically, certification in death education is offered through the Association for Death Education and Counseling (ADEC). Most hospice programs have a health care professional in this role. This person may be a nurse, counselor, or social worker. The Medicare hospice regulations require an organized bereavement program under the supervision of qualified personnel.[2] Bereavement services are provided up to one year after the death of the patient. The functions of the bereavement counselor are listed in Table 4–8. Bereavement is a process that occurs following the death of a person with whom one has shared a significant relationship. Grief is the emotional response to bereavement while mourning is the physical expression of grief. There is a psychosocial transition which follows bereavement where a person's place in their world is suddenly altered. It is during this transition period when a bereavement counselor is of great value in assisting the family members through their phases of grief.[13] It is essential to recognize individuals and families at risk for complicated bereavement, such as unresolved emotional entanglements. Bereavement outcomes in the first few months after a death must encompass a continuum of experiences which include a physical, emotional, social, and spiritual component.[14] It is often helpful to encourage bereaved family members to attend bereavement support groups where expression of grief and loss can be safely displayed and support and acknowledgement may be received. Bereavement groups are not designed to function as therapy groups; discussion of deep inner issues is not encouraged. If possible, it is best to run groups which bring together people with similar experiences, for example parents who have lost a child. Many hospices use volunteer bereavement counselors to lead the group. While this practice has certainly proven helpful, licensed staff should consistently monitor the group to provide guidance and support. Memorial services are often arranged as quarterly or annual events. Hospice staff and bereaved families join together to commemorate the dead. Symbolic ritual can often assist the process of closure.

TABLE 4–8    Functions of a Bereavement Counselor

Assist team members in identifying individuals at risk for complicated bereavement by developing assessment tools, interventions, and referral patterns

Assist the interdisciplinary team members with bereavement issues

Develop and facilitate bereavement support groups

Coordinate and facilitate memorial services for bereaved families

Establish training goals for interdisciplinary team members concerning grief issues

Work within and contribute to an interdisciplinary team

## *Other Counselors*

The Medicare hospice regulations require dietary and any other counseling services be available to individuals and their families.[2] The majority of nutritional counseling is related to loss of appetite and may be done by the nurse. However, there may be times when a nutritionist is asked to consult on a particularly complex problem. Medicare does not require specific training or certification. Therefore, hospice programs must recruit counselors with appropriate education and experience, and provide them with additional training. Lay persons and professionals may fill the counselor role.

## ❖ Summary

Clearly, the interdisciplinary team members must work well in a group and be committed to a give-and-take collaborative process of care. Although each member will bring his or her own expertise, perspective, and life experiences to bear, there will also be a certain amount of role blurring. They may be called upon to play a role in which they have not had formal training. For example, the nurse may serve as spiritual advisor or the chaplain as clinical observer. It will be up to the team member to assess the situation, provide as much care as each is able in the immediate circumstance, and then refer to the appropriate team member for further assistance. When the interdisciplinary team members work well together, the result is synergistic for the patient, the family, and the hospice caregivers.

## ❖ References

1. Cassell, E.J. "The Nature of Suffering and the Goals of Medicine." *New England Journal of Medicine,* 306:639–645, 1982.
2. *Medicare: Hospice Manual.* U.S. Department of Health and Human Services. U.S. Department of Commerce National Technical Information Service, Washington, DC, 1992.

3. MacDonald, N. "Oncology and Palliative Care: The Case for Co-ordination." *Cancer Treatment Reviews, 19*(Supplement A):29–41, 1993.

4. Levy, M.H. "Integration of Pain Management into Comprehensive Cancer Care." *Cancer, 63*:2328–2335, 1989.

5. World Health Organization. *Cancer Pain Relief and Palliative Care.* Geneva: World Health Organization, 1990.

6. Eng, M.A. "The Hospice Interdisciplinary Team: A Synergistic Approach to the Care of Dying Patients and Their Families." *Holistic Nursing Practice, 7*(6):49–56, 1993.

7. Johanson, G.A. *Physician's Handbook of Symptom Relief in Terminal Care.* Santa Rosa, CA: Sonoma County Academic Foundation for Excellence in Medicine, 1988.

8. Dobratz, M.C. "Hospice Nursing: Present Perspectives and Future Directives." *Cancer Nursing, 13*(2):116–122, 1990.

9. Dicks, B. "The Contribution of Nursing to Palliative Care." *Palliative Medicine,* 197–203, 1990.

10. Knight, C.F., and Knight, P.F. "Developing a Certificate Course for Hospice Nurses: A Delphi Survey of Subject Areas." *Hospice Journal, 8*(3):45–57, 1992.

11. Amenta, M. "Certification for Hospice Nurses? Assessment of Need." *Hospice Journal, 8*(3):73–87, 1992.

12. Dunlop, R.J., and Hockley, J.M. *Terminal Care Support Teams.* Oxford: Oxford University Press, 1990.

13. Billings, J.A. *Outpatient Management of Advanced Cancer.* Philadelphia: Lippincott Co., 1985.

14. Mor, V., Greer, D.S., and Kastembaum. R., eds. *The Hospice Experiment.* Baltimore: John Hopkins University Press, 1988.

# ❖ Chapter 5
# Additional Team Members

LISA SZCZEPANIAK

In this chapter we will describe the members of the hospice care team other than those defined as core team members. We have divided them into three groups: essential team members, additional team members, and the office staff including administrative staff. Essential team members are those who must be available to meet the needs of the patient. According to the Medicare hospice regulations home health aides, homemakers, and office staff may provide services by contract arrangements with the hospice program.[1] Volunteers must be hired directly by the hospice program. Therefore, the team members are determined by each patient's needs at any given point in time. This is in contrast to the core services, described in Chapter 4, that are part of every patient's care plan. Bunn notes that volunteers are the backbone of hospice.[2] The Medicare hospice regulations consider volunteers as employees of the hospice who must provide a minimum of five percent of the patient care hours.

## ❖ Essential Team Members

### *Home Health Aide/Homemaker*

A survey conducted by The Foundation for Hospice and Home Care in 1986 found that there were twelve different commonly used names in the United States to describe paraprofessionals who provide health and supportive services.[3] The most appropriate names to describe these individuals in hospice are homemaker or home health aide. Table 5–1 lists the elements important to the qualifications and responsibilities of the homemaker/home health aide.

Home health aides play a vital role in the care of the dying patient because they are the team members who are in the patient's home most frequently and who usually experience the home situation most intensely. Creating an intensive selection, orientation, support, and evaluation process for home health aides assists in their retention and success.[4] During the selection process, it is necessary to consider candidates with home health aide experience, preferably hospice home care. There may be times when a home health aide has personal experience caring for a dying patient or family member. This experience may give the candidate the ability to understand the hospice philosophy and approach to care.

41

TABLE 5–1   Job Description: Home Health Aide/Homemaker

| Qualifications | Responsibilities |
| --- | --- |
| Empathetic communication skills | Observe, report, and document patient status and care promptly |
| Respect for patient's privacy and property | |
| Positive attitude | Read and record temperature, pulse, and respirations |
| Flexible | Maintain clean, safe environment |
| Dependable | Perform appropriate and safe techniques in personal hygiene and grooming |
| Reliable | |
| Good observation skills | Perform safe transfer techniques |
| Understanding of team approach and limit setting | Perform normal range of motion and positioning |
| High school diploma or equivalent | Assist in healthy meal preparation |
| One year homemaker or hospice experience | Assist patients to self-administer medications |
| Ability to work within and contribute to an interdisciplinary team | Light housekeeping |

The responsibilities of the home health aide include providing personal care to patients and respite to caregivers. They may assist the patient in administering their medications and preparing healthy meals. The home health aide is responsible for light housekeeping, providing a safe environment, and reporting changes in the patient's status promptly to the primary nurse. It is necessary for the home health aide to attend interdisciplinary team meetings to communicate with all team members on a regular basis.

The orientation, support, and evaluation processes are vital to the success of the home health aide.[5] Orientation and support begin on the first day. Expectations should be clearly outlined in the job description. The expectations of the home health aide as a team member should be discussed in the context of hospice philosophy and care. The importance of communication and team interaction should be emphasized. The roles of all team members should be reviewed as well as the hospice mission statement, history, funding, and organizational culture in an effort to assist new employees to understand their roles within the organization. It is also important that the home health aide understands what occurs during the initial referral, case opening, the initiation of the interdisciplinary plan of care, interdisciplinary team meetings, the role of each team member in the home, and the bereavement process. With this knowledge, the home health aide can comprehend the hospice concept and their own role in the program.

Proficiency of skills is often evaluated during the orientation process. The supervisor demonstrates the specific skill and then observes a return demonstration by the aide. A specific skill may need to be reviewed before proficiency can be documented. The skills test should be repeated at least every twelve months. Medicare hospice regulations require the primary nurse to supervise the home health aide. A list of important home health aide skills is presented in Table 5–2.

The home health aide's first home visit alone is sometimes stressful. Appropriate information, support, and guidance will help to ease the stress. A written plan of care should be prepared for the home health aide by the primary nurse. It is imperative to discuss the patient's physical needs and home situation with all the team members involved in the case prior to the first visit. It can be overwhelming for the home health aide to enter a difficult situation in the home without prior knowledge of the situation.

Home health aides provide intimate personal care to their patients. This may be a time when patients reveal their deepest feelings. During the orientation process, it is important to teach the home health aide basic communication skills, encourage open communication between team members, and assist the aide in meeting the patient's needs.

The role of the home health aide can be very challenging. A typical day may include a meeting in the office, followed by three to four home visits to assist in personal care. Some of the patients may be actively dying and need personal care as well as emotional support. The family may need support and guidance in providing comfort measures. The personal care for hospice patients is very involved with most patients requiring total care. The home health aide may share a special bond with patients and their families because of the amount of time spent in the homes. Moreover, since the aide spends less time in the office and more time in the patient's home, it is vital to be aware of their level of stress and provide support. The information that the home health aide shares with the team is integral to a comprehensive plan of care. As a member of the interdisciplinary team, the aide can participate in team conferences, mini-team conferences, and support groups. They receive informal support from other team members and give support when needed.

TABLE 5–2   Home Health Aide Skills

Complete bed bath and linen change

Bowel and bladder care
(e.g., digital rectal examination to check for fecal impaction, ostomy care, Foley catheter care)

Skin care
(e.g., simple dressings, decubitus ulcer care)

Backrub

Active and passive range of motion

Transfer techniques

Personal grooming
(e.g., shaving, shampooing, oral hygiene)

Safety measures
(e.g., oxygen safety, during seizures, environmental)

## Physical Therapist, Occupational Therapist, Speech Therapist

The Medicare hospice regulations mandate these services for symptom control or to enable the patient to maintain activities of daily living and basic functional skills. They are usually consultants to the team. Their work is directed toward maintaining or enhancing function and quality of life rather than rehabilitation. The physical therapist may teach active and passive range of motion as well as transfer techniques from bed to chair. The occupational therapist may evaluate the need for built-up eating utensils in a patient with severe arthritis. The speech pathologist may teach swallowing or communication techniques to a patient with amyotrophic lateral sclerosis. These are just a few of the many ways these therapists interact with the interdisciplinary team.

## Volunteer

Volunteers are vital members of the team. Briggs suggests that most hospice organizations rely heavily on volunteers to provide many hospice services.[6] Patients, families, and the interdisciplinary team have a variety of needs. People have many reasons for volunteering. One survey reported that the most important reasons individuals volunteered were to help others or repay others for their own good fortune and religious beliefs. Many individuals become hospice volunteers because they had a good experience with hospice or someone close to them died alone in pain.

Hospice programs employ volunteer coordinators to facilitate volunteer recruitment, orientation, and assignments. This person may represent the volunteers in the interdisciplinary team meeting, although volunteers are encouraged to attend meetings when their patients are presented. The volunteer coordinator is a source of support and guidance for the volunteers.

Hospice volunteers share many characteristics. The first is empathy, which is defined as putting oneself in another's place in order to understand him or her better. A second characteristic is being comfortable with dying patients and their families. Paradis and Usu state that these characteristics combined with minimal anxiety and caring will not predict success in a volunteer.[7] They suggest that a volunteer's success is predicted by traits such as comfortableness with death, motivation, involvement in other community activities, and availability.

Volunteers care for individuals and their families in a variety of ways. Some of these include direct personal care through bed baths, toileting, shampoos, and exercise. Volunteers provide support by reassuring, consoling, listening, and assisting in life review. The volunteer may entertain the patient and family by sharing jokes, playing music, working together on hobbies, and reading. Spiritual support is also very important in the role of spiritual care volunteer. The volunteer may discuss spiritual issues, assist in prayer, and listen to fears of death and dying. Many volunteers assist in light housekeeping, vacuuming, laundry, and running errands. Volunteers can provide support to the caregivers by providing respite, thereby giving the family a break from caregiving. Volunteers may also work in the hospice office. They can assist with filing and billing, answer the telephone, enter data into the computer, help with correspondences, and order and organize medical and office supplies. Volunteers may serve as fundraisers, board members, and consultants.[8]

Many hospice programs include volunteer training sessions in the orientation of all new hospice employees, paid staff, and volunteers. These sessions include presentations on the hospice philosophy and mission, the interdisciplinary team concept, and the roles of the team members. Pain and symptom management issues are presented in basic terms to assist the volunteer in understanding the disease process. Personal care may be provided by some volunteers and is therefore a part of the training program. Discussions regarding family dynamics, alcohol and substance abuse, and therapeutic communication provide the volunteer with the knowledge needed to identify situations that may potentially affect the safety of the patient. New hospice workers are presented with procedures for communicating their concerns to other team members.

## *Pharmacist*

The pharmacist is specially trained and holds a Bachelor of Science degree in pharmacy. This individual is also registered with the state board of pharmacy. The pharmacist may be registered in several states. Just as each patient comes to hospice with his or her own attending physician, the patient may also choose a pharmacist. If the patient is enrolled in one of the managed care options (e.g., Medicare hospice benefit), the choice must be made from a list of pharmacies with which the hospice has contracts. It is important for one pharmacy to fill all of the patient's prescriptions so that polypharmacy can be monitored. The pharmacist also monitors the patient's medication profile for allergies, drug/drug and food/drug interactions. The pharmacist is a valuable resource for the nurse, physician, patient, and family.

## ❖ Additional Team Members

### *Expressive Therapies*

Expressive therapies are also known as creative arts. They include music, art, drama, dance, poetry, and writing. The emphasis of these therapies is placed on personal contact and the value of the individual as a creative person.[9] An individual may use the arts as a vehicle to discuss memories and associations which arise from the creative process. Life review may encompass places, friends, work experiences, and meaningful life events. The arts serve to stimulate the senses. Music and the spoken word provide auditory stimulation. Paintings, photographs, or a vase full of beautiful flowers provide visual stimulation. Tactile stimulation may be found in petting a dog, receiving a soothing backrub or holding a special hand. The olfactory sense may be stimulated by fragrant flowers, seasonal greens, or the aroma of freshly baked bread.[10] Music and art therapists are sometimes employed by hospice programs. Their roles will be discussed in more detail.

## Music Therapist

Music therapy is the intentional use of music as a form of psychological or spiritual support or as an adjunct to symptom management and nursing care. The music therapist is specially trained and professionally accredited. Several colleges and universities in the United States offer Bachelor and Master of Arts degrees in music therapy. These academic programs include didactic work as well as 1,040 hours of supervised clinical work. The music therapist may become board certified by successfully passing a test offered by the Certification Board for Music Therapists, thereby earning the credentials RMT-BC or CMT-BC. The credentials are dependent on whether the college or university is affiliated with The National Association of Music Therapy (RMT-BC) or The American Association of Music Therapy (CMT-BC). The music interventions used by the music therapist are based on a wide knowledge of music, behavioral sciences, current treatment, educational and medical models, and accepted therapeutic approaches. The interplay of relationships between the patient, the music, and the therapist is integral to the treatment plan.[11] The music interventions are designed to meet the needs of the patient and/or family. Some examples include listening to music, composing songs for family members, using specific sounds to promote relaxation, and combining music and visual imagery to promote relaxation. The music therapist may help the patient to explore sounds which remind him/her of a restful place. These sounds are then combined with the therapist's voice to make a guided imagery audiotape which is specific to the patient. The acronym CRISP has been developed by two music therapists to assist with the planning and intervention phases of music therapy in the hospice population. They use CRISP to structure their clinical notes. The details of CRISP are outlined in Table 5–3.[12] Hospice programs may have a music therapist on staff or the therapist may be a consultant to the team. Most music therapists are reimbursed by the hospice program. However, some private practitioners have been successful in obtaining reimbursement from third party payers.

## Art Therapist

Art therapy is used to assist the patient, family, and team members to explore their feelings and provides a vehicle for expression. It is used with adults as well as children. Art media can be especially helpful in

TABLE 5–3    CRISP Music Therapy

C    Composition (songwriting, instrumental composition)

R    Relaxation techniques

I    Improvisation (structured and unstructured composition)

S    Singing

P    Playing an instrument

*Sources:* Katherine Ryan, RMT-BC, and Brenda Calovini, MA, RMT-BC (personal interview).

providing a more comfortable, less threatening mode of expression than verbal communication.[13] Individuals may express themselves artistically through painting, sculpture, designing masks, jewelry, or collages. The opportunities are as endless as the imagination. The art therapist is specially trained. Some colleges and universities in the United States offer a Master of Arts degree in art therapy. The individual may become a registered art therapist (ATR) after 1,000 hours of supervised clinical work. Currently, there is no third party reimbursement for art therapy.

## Respiratory Therapist

The respiratory therapist is specially trained. This individual must complete a certification program and the specific requirements vary from state to state. The new graduate must pass a licensing test which leads to the credentials CRTT (certified respiratory therapist technician). The respiratory therapist is often consulted regarding the appropriate use of liquid oxygen, humidification, oxygen concentrators, and liter flow. The respiratory therapist is often employed by a supplier with whom the hospice has a contract. The therapist may consult with the physician or nurse in this position.

## Medical Specialists

Any of the medical specialists may be asked to consult with the team regarding a specific problem. This is usually done in collaboration with the hospice medical director and the attending physician. An anesthesiologist may be asked to perform a celiac plexis block for a patient with intractable pain due to pancreatic cancer. A surgeon may be asked to insert a PEG tube for a patient with an esophageal obstruction. A psychiatrist may be asked to evaluate a patient for depression. A clinical psychologist may be asked to assist with complex bereavement issues.

## Other Consultants

The list of possible consultants is endless. The Medicare hospice regulations mandate an ongoing program for the training of hospice employees. There are many options for inservices and workshops for staff and volunteers. These may include pain and symptom management, team building, the development of a quality assurance program, and cultural diversity. Hospices may hire consultants to develop and provide educational programs. Other consultants may include individuals to write grant proposals, experts in computer program development, public relations consultants, and community leaders.

## ❖ The Office Staff as Team Members

### Hospice Managers

The executive director is responsible for the vision and direction of the hospice program. The management staff work together to develop goals and objectives for the program. They must define what is needed and who will be involved in the work. The managers involve their staff in the planning and implementation phases of the work. Staff involvement is integral to the success of any hospice program.

### Office Staff

The members of the office staff play a vital role in the daily operations of the hospice program. The three most common roles are medical records clerk, clerical, and receptionist. To perform successfully, the office staff should meet the following minimum requirements: a high school diploma, knowledge of medical terms, word processing skills, experience in a medical office setting, and basic understanding of the hospice concept. These are vital roles because they provide continuity of record-keeping and communication between the hospice staff, family, and patients. Finally, they are a resource for the information necessary to successfully carry out the mission of the hospice program.

## ❖ Summary

The information presented here is offered as a guide to recruiting, orienting, and retaining interdisciplinary team members. The team approach can be challenging and requires much work and energy to create a highly synergistic team.

## ❖ References

1. U.S. Department of Health and Human Services. *Medicare: Hospice Manual*. Washington, DC: U.S. Department of Commerce National Technical Information Service, 1992.
2. Bunn, E. "Volunteers as the Backbone . . ." *Caring*, 4(2):19–20, 1985.
3. Training and Certification of Homemaker-Home Health Aides. Foundation for Hospice and Homemaker and National Association for Home Care. *Caring*, 9(4):31–38, 1990.

4. Tomczyk, M. "Preparing Homemaker-Home Health Aides to Care for Hospice Clients." *Caring,* 9(11):18–21, 1990.
5. Stephany, T. "Hospice Home Health Aides." *Home Healthcare Nurse,* 2:71, 1993.
6. Briggs, J. "Volunteer Qualities: A Survey of Hospice Volunteers." *Oncology Nursing Forum,* 14(1):27–31, 1987.
7. Paradis, L., and Usui, W. "Hospice Volunteers: The Impact of Personality Characteristics on Retention and Job Performance." *Hospice Journal,* 3(1):3–30, 1987.
8. Stephany, T. "Identifying Roles of Hospice Volunteers." *Home Healthcare Nurse,* 7(3):51–52, 1989.
9. Aldridge, D. "Hope, Meaning and the Creative Art Therapies in the Treatment of AIDS." *The Arts in Psychotherapy,* 20:285–297, 1993.
10. Orser, A. M. "The Creative Arts in the Hospice Setting." *Thanatos,* 9:9–15, Fall 1991.
11. Porchet-Munro, S. "Music Therapy." In *Oxford Textbook of Palliative Medicine,* D. Doyle, G.W.C. Hanks, and N. MacDonald, eds. Oxford: Oxford University Press, 1993.
12. Ryan, K. Personal communication. *Hospice of the Western Reserve,* Cleveland, OH.
13. Krug, C. "Art Therapy with the Terminally Ill in a Hospice Setting." Ursuline College, 1993.

## ❖ For Further Reading

Mandel, S.E. "Music Therapy: Variations on a Theme." *Journal of Palliative Care,* 9(4):37–55, 1993.

Marcant, D., and Rapin, C.H. "Role of the Physiotherapist in Palliative Care." *Journal of Pain and Symptom Management,* 8(21):68–71, 1993.

Munro, S., and Mount, B. "Music Therapy in Palliative Care." *Canadian Medical Association Journal,* 9:1029–1034, 1978.

Paradis, L., Miller, B., and Runnion, V. "Volunteer Stress and Burnout: Issues for Administration." *Hospice Journal,* 3(2–3):223–253, 1987.

Welk, T. "The Hospice Volunteer: A Person of Hospitality." *American Journal of Hospice and Palliative Care,* 9(4):9–10 1992.

West, T.M. "Psychological Issues in Hospice Music Therapy." *Music Therapy Perspectives,* 12(2):117–124, 1994.

Zimmerman, L., Pozehl, B., Duncan, K., and Schmitz, R. "The Effects of Music in Patients Who Had Chronic Pain." *Western Journal of Nursing Research,* 11:298–309, 1989.

# ❖ Chapter 6

# Hospice Care Settings

BETTY L. SCHMOLL

CAROL E. DIXON

In the 1970s, hospice care developed in response to concerns about care for terminally ill patients. When asked, most people preferred to die at home—and yet most deaths were occurring in acute care hospitals. In general, both the setting and the care did not address the broader needs of terminally ill patients and their families. It seemed clear that something different was needed. Community groups began exploring ways to develop holistic care for people with life-threatening illnesses and their families. From the beginning, hospice programs were developed based on the premise that health care should be patient-driven and consumer-oriented. The nature, structure, and function of hospices were shaped by the belief that the care of dying individuals should be grounded in human values and the primary goal of hospice care should be to keep patients in the familiar surroundings of their own homes as long as possible and appropriate. The frustration of trying to access necessary resources to provide care to the terminally ill in a medical model health care system influenced the structure of hospice licensure laws and the development of the Medicare hospice benefit.[1]

There has been an expansion and enrichment of what hospice can do and a formalization and redefinition of hospice care. The current definition of hospice care is still a concept of care, but this has been expanded to include a distinct, comprehensive cluster of services for terminally ill individuals and their families that are provided on a continuum of intensity (levels of care) in a variety of care settings. The services which are required under the Medicare Hospice Regulations are listed in Table 2–7. It is important to note that specific services are based on the patient's individualized plan of care.

## ❖ Service Mix

All hospice care includes access to and availability of appropriate and necessary services to meet the identified needs and choices for care made by the patient and family. The Medicare hospice benefit Conditions of Participation define a distinctive cluster of services that the hospice must provide regardless of the care setting.[1] It also establishes qualifications for how hospice care is provided. These are discussed in Chapter 2.

## ❖ Levels of Care

Four levels of care are identified in the Medicare hospice regulations.[1] They are listed in Table 6–1.

ROUTINE HOME CARE, the most common level of care, is the heart of hospice care. The full scope of hospice services is provided by the hospice team, most often in the patient's personal residence. Care begins with an admission process which includes an assessment and evaluation of the patient's status and appropriateness for hospice care. During the initial visit, the focus is on discovering the concerns and issues that are troubling the patient and family and in helping them understand what hospice care is and how it can help. Frequently, care during the first few visits is directed toward relieving specific problems such as pain, symptoms of the disease, or anxiety. From the assessment visit on, the patient and family are evaluated for the need of specific services, supplies, equipment, and community resources. This initial attention to the needs of the patient and family are a pattern for continuing re-evaluation. Patient and family needs and concerns are continually being re-appraised to ensure that support and comfort-oriented services, appropriate and necessary for the palliation and support of the patient and family, are offered in a timely manner. In routine home care, there is usually significant involvement of family or primary care support persons providing direct, hands-on care for the patient. This care can be quite complex, and teaching and support for the caregiver is an important part of hospice care. By meeting the comfort needs of the patient and the support needs of the family, many patients are able to die, as they prefer, at home.

CONTINUOUS HOME CARE is an expanded level of care in the home. It allows up to twenty-four hours a day of skilled nursing to ease patients through periods of crisis and to prevent hospitalization for management of acute symptoms. Although the chief reason for this level of care is management of acute physical symptoms, it may also be used when the burden of caregiving for families is greater than their resources. Usually this occurs because care of the patient is complex, difficult, or extensive. There are no limits to the number of hours or days allowed at this level, but care must be primarily skilled nursing for at least eight hours out of twenty-four to qualify. Hours need not be consecutive, nor does all of the care need to be provided by a registered nurse. However, at least one hour more than half the total continuous home care hours must be provided by a registered

TABLE 6–1    Levels of Care

Routine home care

Continuous home care

Respite care

Regular inpatient care

nurse or licensed practical nurse. Continuous home care provides an invaluable resource for helping patients to stay at home—and die at home.

RESPITE CARE supports the patient's family and caregivers. They need time away from the intensity of caring for a terminally-ill individual. Respite care is designed to give families and caregivers a five-day break from caregiving. Families can plan a mini-vacation, attend special events, or simply get much needed rest and recreation at home while the patient is cared for in an inpatient setting. Respite care is provided for five-day periods by hospices in either their own facilities or contracted beds in nursing homes or hospitals. Care is very similar to homecare except that room and board and assistance with basic activities of living by nurses and nursing assistants are provided in an inpatient setting to replace the care usually provided by the family and caregivers. Respite care must be provided in a Medicare-certified facility. The episodes of respite care must be intermittent, relatively infrequent, and limited to five-day periods. These patients are often very ill or have significant need for assistance with activities of daily living (ADL), which is often the precipitating factor in the family's need for respite care. The typical needs of the patient who requires respite care are expensive due to the intensity of care. The staffing and support required for this level of care usually far exceed the reimbursement for the service.

REGULAR INPATIENT CARE is something of a misnomer. It would be better labeled *Symptom Management* or *Acute Care* because it actually is a substitute for acute care hospitalization. Admission for regular inpatient care is primarily related to medical problems requiring nursing and medical management. Typical problems requiring regular inpatient care are outlined in Table 6–2. In general, any patient whose care is so complex or demanding that the family can no longer continue to provide homecare is a candidate for regular inpatient care. The most noticeable similarity between hospitalization and regular inpatient care is primarily in the skilled nursing and medical management of the patient. The major differences are the focus on palliation of symptoms, the complexity of hospice team services provided, the attention to the family, and the psychosocial and spiritual support that are prevalent in hospice care. Palliative care is designed to provide comfort and support rather than cure of the illness or the problem. There is a limit to the number of inpatient care days a hospice can provide under the Medicare hospice benefit.[1] At least 80 percent of all patient care days must be home care days, and no more than 20 percent of days can be spent in the combination of respite and regular inpatient care. The limitation on inpatient days has not created a problem for hospices since few hospices exceed 7 percent of their program days in inpatient care levels.

## ❖ New Levels of Care

Residential Care, Day Care, and Extended Caregiver Programs (also called In-Home Respite) are relatively new additions to hospice care.

TABLE 6–2    Acute Care Criteria

Imminent death under specific conditions

Bleeding—active and potential

Sepsis

Seizures

Impending delirium tremens

Uncontrolled pain

Any uncontrolled symptom

Central nervous system dysfunction—delirium, coma, dementia

Fractures of weight-bearing bones

Management of complex medications

Acute cardiac symptoms—myocardial infarction, arrhythmias

Complex treatment schedule requiring frequent dressing changes or procedures that require the time, skill, and observations of a professional nurse

Terminal agitation

They are not included in the Medicare hospice benefit as separate levels of care. They are being provided to expand services to meet identified patient care needs. There are charges for these services, usually based on a sliding scale. Charges are frequently waived for indigent patients. Some hospices operate these optional programs with grant money from foundations or from special fund raising projects.

RESIDENTIAL CARE is provided in hospice inpatient settings for patients who require supportive care related to safety needs, weakness, or the inability to perform self-care. It was developed in response to the Medicare hospice benefit's limit on regular inpatient care and the need to provide inpatient care for patients without caregivers or for those whose caregivers are frail, elderly, or fatigued by the intensity of care. Other patients who utilize residential care have caregivers who must work to ensure continued health insurance coverage and family income. Residential care also provides a way to offer better continuity for those patients who are no longer appropriate for regular inpatient care status, but require supportive care related to safety needs, weakness, or the inability to perform self-care for those who do not have an able caregiver to help them. In defining criteria for residential care admission, the norm is patients whose care can safely be provided by a nursing assistant with minimal supervision. This helps to differentiate between regular inpatient and residential care patients. If the patient's condition changes so that a more intensive level is needed, the hospice can transfer the patient to a regular inpatient or continuous home care level to meet the care needs. Residential care is provided in hospice facilities or in contracted beds in hospitals or nursing homes. In either case, the hospice is responsible to ensure that care and services meet hospice standards.

DAY CARE is relatively new to hospice in the United States. It is designed to provide relief to the caregiver and diversive activities for the patient. It is similar to other adult day care programs for patients with specific health care problems. Patients are transported to the day care site by family or by the hospice. There are planned activities, meals, and observation and assistance as needed. Day care is not easily used by very ill and debilitated patients. This has tended to slow the development of day care programs in hospice settings. Recently, some hospice programs have extended hospice day care to "pre-hospice" patients and their families as a way to familiarize them with hospice care.

EXTENDED CAREGIVER SERVICES or In-Home Respite Care, is a new level which is growing in popularity in hospice programs. The term describes a program that offers shifts of nursing assistants to a patient to supplement or substitute for family caregivers. The goal is to keep the patient at home. Extended caregiver service is needed and used by working families, and frail caregivers, and in situations where the physical demands for caregiving are beyond the strength of the caregiver. It is also a way to supplement care when residential care beds are not immediately available. It is possible to use extended caregiver programs, where extra help in the home is offered to supplement the family's care for patients whose temporary needs cannot easily or appropriately be satisfied through regular homecare or inpatient services. This is an optional service some hospices provide when they are able to fund the care through special fund raising projects, community support, or foundation grants. Although extended caregiver service is not a mandated level of care, it is important to remember that other required levels of care must be available to hospice patients. There are financial and staffing limitations to hospices' ability to provide these new services. These added levels of care have become a valuable extension to hospice services. Because of the extra support available, hospice has been able to provide additional services to individuals and their families.

## ❖ Service Settings

Hospice care is defined not only by services and levels of care provided, but also by the settings in which these services are delivered. Care in the patient's personal residence is always routine home care or continuous home care. Care in a facility can and does include any of the levels of care provided by hospice: routine home care, continuous home care, residential care, day care, respite care, and regular inpatient care.[1]

### Home

What is home? The National Hospice Organization, in its *Standards of a Hospice Program of Care* simply defines home as "a person's place of residence."[2] This definition includes a variety of settings that, at first glance, do not seem to be "home." Hospice home care is being provided in all these settings—adult foster care homes, congregate living and group homes, AIDS housing, hospice residences, tents, homeless shelters, jails, nursing homes, and many other kinds of personal residence imaginable. The commonality in this care is the services provided by hospice, and the responsibility that hospice has to ensure the safety and comfort of the patient, the patient's family, and the hospice staff.

## Facility-Based Care

When care is provided in a facility, regardless of the level of care provided, hospice has a professional management responsibility for the safety and comfort of the patient. This may be a more significant responsibility than in the patient's home since care is being provided by paid caretakers rather than family. Currently there are few rules for residential or nursing home care to ensure quality care and appropriate services. The National Hospice Organization's *Standards of a Hospice Program of Care* and the Medicare Hospice Regulations provide basic guidelines for this care.[2,3] The Medicare Hospice Regulations will undoubtedly expand and develop specific "rules" in the future. Currently, the basic requirements include hospice's responsibility for ensuring that the scope of services is adequate to meet the needs of the patient. The services must be of the same quality and volume to ensure comfort and safety. Hospice staff are expected to meet with the facility's staff to ensure that care is congruent with the hospice plan of care. The hospice retains management oversight responsibility for the patient, and there are some distinct expectations for the care setting that have been established as part of the Medicare hospice benefit guidelines. These reflect hospice values related to facility-based care and include adapting the environment and modifying facility rules to meet the needs of the patient. Adaptation required of the facility are listed in Table 6–3.

TABLE 6–3   Required Facility Adaptation

Ensure privacy and space for family gathering

Allow twenty-four hour visiting and overnight stays

Provide for religious and spiritual worship

Provide flexibility in scheduling care, accommodating individual needs

Permit family to prepare meals

Allow patient choice in food and timing of meals

Provide a comfortable, homelike atmosphere

Ensure access to services required by plan of care

Ensure safety, comfort, and patient satisfaction

Maintain coordination of care by hospice team member

## ❖ Common Service Sites

### *Hospital*

Hospital settings are the most common sites for regular inpatient care, and the most frequent method for providing that care is a "scatter bed" approach. In this model, a hospice contracts with a number of different hospitals in its service area to admit hospice patients for symptom management. The hospice trains hospital staff, develops the plan of care, approves care provided, and pays the hospital for the care. All the usual hospice services are provided with an emphasis on palliation and support for the patient and family. A less common model is the dedicated unit. This is a contracted arrangement with the hospital in which a specific unit or number of beds are reserved for hospice patients. The unit is usually staffed by the hospital, but sometimes the hospice simply rents the space and services of the hospital and staff and operates the unit. It is somewhat easier to control the services provided and ensure appropriate care in this model than in the scatter bed approach since hospice staff are in more direct contact with the patient and better able to control the care provided. A disadvantage of the hospital setting for hospice care is the difficulty in controlling the care provided in a setting owned and operated by another health care provider. In the hospital environment it is easy to access invasive, curative interventions; this availability can create a problem for the hospice in ensuring palliative and comfort-oriented care. A patient may refuse to use a particular hospital for various reasons such as convenience, family preference, religious or philosophical perspectives, or because of their physician's privileges or preferences. The financial and logistical advantages of the hospital setting more than offset the disadvantages, and the hospital setting continues to be the dominant inpatient service setting. Occasionally, hospices also provide respite care in hospitals, but this is rare because the reimbursement level for respite care is too low to be appealing to many hospitals.

### *Long-Term Care Facility*

Nursing homes are used as sites for regular inpatient care, respite care, and routine home care. Reimbursement and the ability to offer expanded care for residents are inducements to the nursing home to contract with the hospice. The favorable surroundings, lower cost of contracting for regular inpatient and respite care, and the ability to increase their patient census are benefits for the hospice. The differences between long-term care regulations and hospice regulations require careful negotiation and ongoing cooperation between nursing home and hospice staff. The nursing home must be Medicare certified, and the hospice requirement that a registered nurse be on the premises and available to provide hands-on care twenty-four hours a day can create a problem for the nursing facility. There is a growing trend for hospices to provide care in extended care facilities. Dedicated beds or dedicated units for regular inpatient and respite care are a familiar part of hospice inpatient care. Routine home care offered in nursing homes is a more recent and growing part of hospice care. It requires the same level and mix of services provided to other hospice home care patients, and it can be an equally valuable resource to terminally ill patients in nursing homes. There have not yet been specific guidelines established for routine home care in nursing home settings; there is a growing concern that some way to ensure the quality of hospice care in nursing homes needs to be developed. It is quite probable that Medicare will develop some measurable guidelines in the near future.

## Hospice Facilities

In the early days of hospice, there was no reimbursement or licensure for hospice care. As a result, the first hospice facilities developed were licensed as specialty hospital hospices, nursing homes, or extended care facilities, and the level of care they could offer was limited to regular inpatient care. The difficulty with this classification was that the licensure requirements which applied specifically to those facilities were inappropriate for hospice care. In addition, the cost of meeting those requirements increased the cost to hospices for providing inpatient care. When the Medicare hospice benefit was enacted, the reimbursement level for inpatient care was much less than the actual cost, and hospices were continually forced to raise funds to keep the facilities operating. The same difficulties were encountered with the development of hospice residences. These facilities were primarily designed to care for home-care patients who needed a sheltered "home" setting. Obtaining licensure for the facility is frequently a long and arduous task, and there is typically no reimbursement for the room and board cost of residential care. Since many hospice patients have very diminished resources to pay for care, fund raising to support the facility once again became a way of life for hospices. Enactment of the Medicare hospice benefit influenced licensure laws and created a reimbursement source for hospice care. The mandate that hospice control the inpatient setting for hospice patient care led to a greater awareness of what quality inpatient care should be and created an incentive for developing a free-standing hospice facility. The broad but clear requirements for "free-standing hospice facilities" meant that hospices could design cost-effective settings to provide acute, residential, and respite care and justify licensure of the facility as a hospice. There are clear advantages to this model. It allows for expeditious transfer of patients from one level of care to another. Since care is provided in the same facility, continuity is enhanced and the need for patients and their families to adapt to new caregivers and new settings is reduced. It ensures both hospice control of the care setting and a consistent pattern of care that meets the hospice's policies and procedures for care. A free-standing hospice facility that provides all levels of care becomes a valuable and important community resource that enhances the hospice's public image and increases access to those who need a variety of levels of care.

## *AIDS Residences*

AIDS residences may be owned and operated by hospices, or they may be community-based homes serving people with AIDS. Comprehensive hospice care is provided in both settings; the primary difference between this and other hospice care is the individual's diagnosis.

## ❖ Summary

Hospice care is a complex mix of interrelationships between services, levels of care, and sites of service. It is the essence of patient-centered, patient-driven, value-based care.

## ❖ References

1. U.S. Department of Health and Human Services. *Medicare: Hospice Manual.*Washington, DC: U.S. Department of Commerce National Technical Information Service, 1992.
2. National Hospice Organization. *Standards of a Hospice Program of Care.* Arlington, VA: National Hospice Organization, 1993.
3. U.S. Department of Health and Human Services. *Interpretive Guidelines—Hospices.* Washington, DC: U.S. Department of Health and Human Services, 1992.

# ❖ Chapter 7

# Quality Care in Hospice

BETTY L. SCHMOLL
CAROL E. DIXON

Attempts to ensure quality health care are as old as the human race's attempts to cure disease. In early cultures, unsuccessful healers were often banished, executed, or permanently maimed by amputating their hands or by inflicting injuries similar to those sustained by their patients. During the 1970s, quality assurance became mandated—it was no longer a voluntary process. The goal was to ensure that all health care providers in the United States met minimum practice standards in an effort to ensure quality care. Recently, the focus of quality assurance has shifted to emphasize patient satisfaction as the critical component of the quality improvement process. Pursuit of quality care is a complex process which demands ongoing commitment. There are no easy formulas or simple instructions which can guarantee patient satisfaction and competent, effective care. Pursuing quality begins with a belief in the value and importance of quality to consumers and to the organization's continued existence. Next it necessitates defining quality and developing an understanding of how various program elements interact to enhance or inhibit quality. Finally, quality practice requires consistent effort, attention to detail, and a commitment of resources. Dr. H. James Harrington, an IBM project quality manager and president of the American Society for Quality Control, defines quality as, "meeting or exceeding customer requirements at a cost that represents value to them." According to Dr. Harrington, excellence is "surpassing customer expectations at a price that represents value to them and delivering consistent performance without repair or excuse."[1]

Translating Dr. Harrington's definition of excellence to hospice practice means surpassing the expectations of patients, families, communities, and regulatory and reimbursement agencies by consistently providing care that is accessible, effective, cost-efficient, supportive, responsive, comforting, and caring. This definition reflects the hospice goal of providing consumer-oriented care and also represents the best of hospice care. How does hospice pursue excellence? It begins with commitment and attention to quality and a desire to improve services and care. Hospice managers explore their own ideas about what constitutes good service and how to measure it. They evaluate performance of similar organizations and review standards established by regulatory and accrediting bodies to identify quality elements to measure and rate their current practice. Deviations from identified "norms" are noted, change or revision in practice is planned and instituted, and the result of the change is evaluated. Then the process begins again. This cyclical recurring process constitutes Continuous Quality Improvement (CQI). Because hospice care is based on the belief that care should be patient-driven and based on patient choice, the patient's response is probably the most meaningful gauge of a hospice's performance. But it is not enough to guarantee quality care and services if other internal and external hospice "customers" are ignored or forgotten. The public's willingness to access hospice services, to cooperate with helping to make those services available, and to provide various resources to enhance the organization's strength and effectiveness stem from confidence in hospice. In addition to patients and their families, hospice's "customers" also include the medical community, funding sources, insurers, staff and volunteers, regulatory and reimbursement agencies, and the general community. It is critical that hospice understands and seeks to satisfy the distinct expectations and dissimilar definitions of value of its many "customers." A hospice's reputation for quality and service is built by demanding quality in every aspect of its operations and structure. This reputation is achieved by ongoing, consistent concern for improvement and a thorough understanding of what constitutes good practice throughout the organization. Quality issues are threaded through the culture, values, and mission of the organization and are reflected in sound management and competent practice. The concept of quality is not static but grows, develops, and matures within the entire organization.

## ❖ Hospice Quality Base

### Board, Management, and the Organization

Concern for quality hospice care is not just the responsibility of staff assigned to quality assurance or quality improvement. It begins and ends with leadership from the board and management of hospice, and it extends to the responsibility each person in the organization has for the quality of his/her own work. Management and board are responsible and accountable for securing adequate resources for the organization and for the wise and appropriate use of those resources. This obligation includes commitment to ensuring the effectiveness and cost-value base of the services provided. Necessary resources means providing sufficient numbers, types, and scope of services to meet the needs of patients and supplying resources to enable staff to offer those services. In reaching toward excellence, sufficient means not just what is provided, but how and when it is provided. Elements of excellence are outlined in Table 7–1.

Frequently, conflicts between the bottom line and service result in efficiency at the expense of meeting human needs. For example, when an organization establishes arbitrary policies that limit or restrict services to simplify

TABLE 7–1   Elements of Excellence

---

Ensuring predictable staffing and services

Establishing fair and equitable policies and procedures to ensure consistent and fair treatment

Providing appropriate equipment, people, and services for efficient performance

Meeting the safety and comfort needs of patients and families

Ensuring care that is timely, responsive, and appropriate

---

management of resources, the result can be "bureaucratic" care that ignores the unique needs of the family. Conversely, the responsibility to allocate resources to get results can be ignored, and the obligation to measure resources spent against results can be forgotten. As an example, a program may need to budget additional monies for a referral coordinator to meet the goal of improving access and maintaining a reputation for timely admissions and response to referrals. The decision to act requires that program managers balance community satisfaction with the improved admission process, more responsive care for the patient and family, and potential financial benefit to the program of earlier admission against the cost of added staff. Financial stability is critical to every organization's survival and hospice is no exception. Without money, there can be no services—thus no potential for quality care. The need to ensure that resources are prudently and efficiently used to meet today's demands must be balanced with the need to ensure adequate resources for the future. Equal attention to both moral and economic issues in allocating funds is critical. Neither can be overemphasized, and neither can be neglected in a quality organization.

Excellence entails more than just a positive bottom line. It includes how and why funds are acquired and spent. Hospice's internal and external customers are keenly interested in how hospice expends its resources. They look for enhancement and expansion of patient care services and for reasonable and appropriate staff salaries and benefits. They expect and want accountability, solvency, and assurance that funds are well-managed and wisely and carefully used to provide service and guarantee survival of the organization. Consistently meeting these expectations is an important measure of program excellence. Ensuring quality throughout the organization means paying attention to every aspect of its function and structure. It includes management responsibility for securing and maintaining safe, comfortable, functional working space for its staff and patients. This necessitates an understanding of the importance of the physical environment. Patient and staff response to care, efficient and harmonious working relationships, and productivity are very directly influenced by the physical setting. For CQI to be effective, hospice needs skilled and competent staff, volunteers and consultants—well-trained, caring people who are committed to patient rights, patient autonomy, and patient choice. Management's obligation to staff extends beyond ensuring safe and appropriate working situations to include suitable salaries and benefits, job-security, and recognition for staff's attention to quality care.

Management must also provide structure, leadership, and guidance to the organization and appropriate support, training, supervision, and resources for staff. Management is further obligated to establish standards for every aspect of the organization and the care delivered by that organization. Policies and procedures that reflect hospice values and ethics for care of the terminally ill are necessary foundation blocks for building and delivering services and are essential for meeting customer expectations. Certain policy areas are particularly relevant to hospice practice. Ensuring access for the variety of people who need and should have care needs consistent attention. Admission and discharge criteria should be regularly evaluated to confirm that they are neither barriers to admission nor blocks for screening out patients. Truth and accuracy in marketing and continual attention to reaching the unserved and underserved are essential to improving access. Management's responsibilities for quality care are outlined in Table 7–2.

## *Care Delivery*

Family caregivers have a key role in hospice care as both customer and provider. The dual role has an enormous impact on the quality of care provided to their family member, the hospice patient. Family members are integral hospice team members. Recognition of their distress and respect for the level of commitment, caring, and sheer hard work involved in caregiving is central to hospice support for the family. Caregivers need reinforcement, support, and education to understand the care needs and to access the many choices for care. Sensitivity to their painful and distressing demands is an important part of providing hospice care. Appreciation and thought for caregivers enhances the family's ability to provide its portion of quality care. Ultimately, services to caregivers and services provided by caregivers are an interrelated aspect of hospice care which significantly influences hospice's

TABLE 7–2  Management's Responsibilities for Quality Care

Ensure a safe work environment

Provide suitable salaries, benefits, and job security

Recognize staff's attention to quality care

Provide structure, leadership, and guidance to the organization

Provide appropriate support, training, supervision, and resources for staff

Establish standards for the organization

Establish policies and procedures that reflect hospice values and ethics reputation for quality. Advocacy for patient's concerns and rights is an important aspect of hospice work. It is important that the role of the caregiver on the hospice team be evaluated as part of CQI. Continuity of care also has special significance in hospice care. Most patients have experienced change and fragmentation of care as they sought specialists and care sites during the preceding months or years of treatment. At a time when their physical and emotional resources are depleted, change is an almost intolerable burden. Quality hospice care requires a commitment to ensuring consistency and continuity in care and care providers. A clear understanding of professional practice standards, education about potential problems, and ongoing supervision to prevent inappropriate and potentially harmful situations from developing is basic to quality practice. For example, staff must understand the narrow line between friendship and a professional relationship and the constant attention necessary to prevent exploiting the gratitude of dying patients and their families. Educating staff about their unique role in patient-family care and the boundaries to that involvement has a significant influence on the quality of hospice care.

## ❖ Hospice Standards

### Regulatory

Licensure laws and Conditions of Participation for the Medicare hospice benefit require hospice programs to monitor and evaluate quality.[2] The evaluation process is not prescribed in these standards, and with the exception of timing and some specific areas to measure, there are few guidelines about the process. Surveys focus on patient satisfaction and compliance with rules related to providing care. Compliance with standards identifies the minimum acceptable practice level and is no guarantee of quality care or service.

### National Hospice Organization (NHO)

NHO, in its recent revision of *Standards for a Hospice Program*, created a comprehensive description of the structure and function of hospice.[3] An accompanying self-assessment tool makes the manual usable by hospices to evaluate their own programs. NHO's goal was to enhance the reliability and credibility of hospice care by providing a guide that hospices' many "customers" could use to identify and/or improve the quality of hospice care. Measuring the structure and performance of the organization set the stage for the development of more definitive, quantitative measures of quality related to service delivery. There has been some concern from hospice providers that patient-outcome measures and "benchmarks" were not part of the revised manual. Establishing outcome measures for hospice must include patient choices and rights, as these are hallmarks of hospice care.

Nevertheless, NHO is currently working on patient-related measurements such as required services and service levels, ethics, and uniform survey tools such as the recent patient-satisfaction survey. NHO is also working to help accrediting bodies design hospice-appropriate standards.

## Joint Commission on Accreditation of Health Care Organizations (JCAHO)

JCAHO had a hospice accreditation program in the past and now plans to include hospice accreditation as part of its revised home health accreditation program. The *1995 Accreditation Manual for Home Care* includes Standards and Scoring Guidelines.[4,5] The accreditation survey will include both direct and contracted services provided by the organization if the organization represents to the public that it provides those services or if the services are provided by "related organizations that are functionally and organizationally integrated with the organization." This could create a problem for hospices since it might require accreditation for hospices that are part of a parent organization accredited by JCAHO unless they seek and are granted a tailored survey. It also means that any organization with which an accredited hospice contracts must also be accredited by or meet existing JCAHO standards for that service. In the next few years, JCAHO expects to redesign their accrediting process and to work toward accrediting health care systems or networks. They plan to accredit services, not providers or organizations. Each health care organization surveyed will specify what it actually does, and appropriate packets of requirements from each of the listed areas would then be used by JCAHO to evaluate and accredit the services provided by that organization. The goal is to accredit every service provided by or purchased by a system or network.

## The National League for Nursing Community Health Accreditation Program (CHAP)

NLN'S CHAP is also currently being revised and updated.[6] CHAP's focus is quality and financial stability as integral to program viability and survivability. Their evaluation program is outlined in Table 7–3. They provide a separate hospice manual with core requirements related to program organization, structure, governance, and function, and a subset of value-based, hospice-specific standards designed to meet Medicare hospice benefit and licensure requirements. The revised manual will include an evaluation section for hospice inpatient care which will broaden the scope of CHAP's accreditation process. CHAP staff are committed to developing an appropriate and comprehensive hospice accreditation program.

TABLE 7–3   CHAP Evaluation Guidelines

---

The organization's structure and function support a consumer oriented philosophy and purpose.

The organization consistently provides high quality services and products.

The organization has adequate human, financial, and physical resources which are effectively organized to accomplish its stated purpose.

The organization is positioned for long-term viability.

---

## ❖ Continuous Quality Improvement (CQI)

CQI (Continuous Quality Improvement) or TQI (Total Quality Improvement) are current terms for quality assurance. The intent is to imply a more intensive and continuing attempt at improvement than in the past. The reality is that new terms are frequently coined to match the problem-solving technique, but new terms do not necessarily mean new practice. Every quality improvement effort follows the same steps—gather data, analyze the information, identify problems, implement a change, and evaluate the results. The goal is also familiar—trying to continually improve outcome. Ideally, CQI should integrate quality assurance, risk-management, infection control, and utilization review into a comprehensive program. It should include all service areas and match both internal and external hospice "customers'" needs for information. Evaluation studies should include: audits/surveys; utilization review; cost containment; staff competency; risk management; and total program evaluation. Table 7–4 outlines a typical CQI program in hospice.

## ❖ Benchmarking

Benchmarking is a current concept that seems to be gaining favor.[7-11] The goal of benchmarking is to measure performance against "the best." It focuses on critical functions and problem areas in order to implement improvement via a continuing process that parallels the problem-solving approach. Benchmarking is a proactive effort to find new ways to enhance the function of the organization. Because it will have an impact on quality, cost, and time efficiency, benchmarking can easily be integrated into a CQI program. Table 7–5 contains a sample of hospice benchmark areas. Benchmarks can be a valuable tool for framing CQI in hospice. They are measures of the organization's overall health and quality which influence the quality of care provided, the reputation of the hospice, the marketability of services, and the survival of the organization.

TABLE 7–4   Hospice CQI Calendar

1. Organization
    Review of data pertaining to use and services—ongoing
    Program evaluation—annual

2. Clinical
    a. Interdisciplinary
        Concurrent and retrospective audits—quarterly
        Team meetings—bi-weekly
        Utilization review—monthly and as needed
        Supervised home visits—annual and as needed
        Staff conferences—monthly and as needed
    b. Medical
        Circumstances of death reviews—monthly
        Review of unusual treatments/procedures—monthly
        Medical management meeting—quarterly and as needed
    c. Special Topics
        Pain control audit—quarterly
        Nutrition evaluation—quarterly
        Nursing home audit—ongoing
        Skin and wound care—quarterly

3. Patient/Family
    Hospice care center audit—quarterly
    Family satisfaction surveys—quarterly

4. Financial
    Financial statements—monthly
    Monitor timing, accuracy, accounts receivable and payable—monthly
    External audit—annual

5. Medical Records
    Completeness—ongoing

6. Staff
    CQC (Comments, Questions, Criticisms)—monthly
    Support services survey—annual
    Employee satisfaction survey—biannual
    Exit interview and survey—ongoing
    Performance appraisal—annual

7. Physicians
    Satisfaction survey—biannual

8. Volunteers
    Satisfaction survey—biannual
    Volunteer phone call survey—current
    Evaluation of volunteers—ongoing

9. Other
    Incident review—monthly
    On call answering service audit—ongoing
    Food service sampling—monthly
    CQI program review—annual

TABLE 7–5   Hospice Benchmark Areas

Patient visits
   Numbers by discipline
   Numbers for on call
   Numbers at patient death

Equipment provided

Medications provided

Charges to patient/family by hospice

Length of stay—patient

Use of levels of care—patient

Restrictions on treatments

Restrictions on admission and retention

Numbers and reasons for discharge

Timeliness of admission after referral is received

Percent of referrals accepted

Cost per patient by insurance type

Mix of services provided

Indigent and charity care

Market penetration

Patient demographics—age, sex, race, diagnosis

Length of stay

## ❖ Summary

Quality is critical to the future of hospice. Tom Hoyer, representing the Health Care Finance Administration (HCFA) at a National Hospice Organization workshop, expressed it well. He said, "If we don't continue to do more than just what is required, we will cease to be unique." It is hospice's unique reputation for doing more than the minimum that has been the foundation for its success.

## ❖ References

1. Harrington, H. J. *The Improvement Process: How America's Leading Companies Improve Quality.* New York: McGraw-Hill, 1976.
2. U.S. Department of Health and Human Services. *Medicare: Hospice Manual, Rev.* Washington, DC: U.S. Department of Commerce National Technical Information Service, 1992.
3. The National Hospice Organization. *Standards of a Hospice Program of Care.* Arlington, VA: The National Hospice Organization, 1993.

4.  Joint Commission on Accreditation of Healthcare Organizations. *1995 Accreditation Manual for Home Care Volume 1. Standards.* Oakbrook Terrace, IL: Joint Commission on Accreditation of Healthcare Organizations, 1994.

5.  Joint Commission on Accreditation of Healthcare Organizations. *1995 Accreditation Manual for Home Care Volume II. Scoring Guidelines.* Oakbrook Terrace, IL. Joint Commission on Accreditation of Healthcare Organizations, 1994.

6.  National League of Nursing. *CHAP STANDARDS—Draft Copy.* New York: National League of Nursing, 1994.

7.  Balm, G. *Benchmarking: A Practitioner's Guide for Becoming and Staying Best of the Best.* Schaumburg, IL: QPMA Press, 1992.

8.  Bogan, C. E., and English, M. J. *Benchmarking for Best Practices: Winning Through Innovative Adaptation.* New York: McGraw-Hill, 1994.

9.  Boxwell, R. J. *Benchmarking for Competitive Advantage.* New York: McGraw-Hill, 1994.

10. Lambertus, T. "Benchmarking the Tool for Dealing with Downsizing, Other Crises." In S. Weakley, ed. *Hospital Benchmarks: The Newsletter of Best Practices.* Atlanta: American Health Consultants, Inc. 1994, 45–50.

11. Spendoline, M. *The Benchmarking Book.* New York: Amacom, 1992.

# ❖ Chapter 8

# Pain Management in the Cancer Patient

WALTER B. FORMAN

DENICE C. SHEEHAN

Pain and symptom management are integral to excellence in the care of the hospice patient. This chapter will present basic information on the management of pain and the next will do the same for other symptoms associated with dying. Sixty to 90 percent of individuals with cancer will have at least one or more "pains" associated with the disease or its treatment.[1] Because many of these individuals have other medical problems (e.g., arthritis), additional causes of pain must be considered. The principle issue in managing cancer-associated pain must begin with clearly identifying each and every pain and its cause before determining the therapy to be prescribed. The hospice professional must be skilled in this assessment. In hospice, total pain assessment includes knowing the related physical, psychosocial, financial, spiritual, and emotional components associated with the pain in order to proceed appropriately.[2] Using current techniques, pain associated with cancer can be managed effectively in up to 95 percent of patients.[3] Many organizations have developed and published guidelines for managing cancer-related pain. They all contain information concerning clinical practice guidelines, education for the patient as well as the professional, ethical concerns, research questions, and administrative issues. The most comprehensive guidelines are available from The Agency for Health Care Policy and Research, Oncology Nursing Society, American Pain Society, World Health Organization, The American Cancer Society, and the State Cancer Pain Initiatives.[4-10] Their addresses can be found in Appendix III.

## ❖ Causes of Pain

Cancer-associated pain can have several clinical patterns. They have been classified by their putative neurophysiological mechanisms.[11] The classifications are nociceptive, including somatic and visceral, and neuropathic. Each produces a classic clinical presentation that must be recognized in order to treat the patient appropriately. Somatic pain is characterized by the individual as stabbing, throbbing, aching, dull, sharp, or cramping. Somatic pain is well localized and is the result of the stimulation of nociceptive receptors. This type of pain is associated with bone metastases, soft tissue infiltration, and post-operative pain. Visceral pain associated with abdominal complaints is often described as a constant ache with intermittant cramping that is poorly localized and often associated with nausea. A primary or metastatic tumor tends to distend, infiltrate, compress, or stretch the thoracic or abdominal viscera. This is common in liver metastases and pancreatic cancer. Visceral pain is often projected to other areas of the body, as for example, left shoulder pain occurring when the diaphragm is irritated in individuals with pancreatic cancer. Neuropathic pain is less common, but clearly a concern when evaluating pain. Usually patients with pain associated with nerve involvement, whether as a result of nerve entrapment or infiltration describe their pain as intermittent burning, lancinating (an electric shock), tingling, and/or shooting into a body area (e.g., into the arm or leg). Peripheral nerves may also be damaged by trauma, radiation, or during chemotherapy (e.g., vinca alkaloids, cisplatin).[12] Neuropathic pain often occurs with mild stimuli such as clothing touching the skin. This phenomena is known as allodynia. Patients who experience neuropathic pain are often extremely distressed because of the noxious nature of the pain.

## Common Misconceptions about Pain

The hospice worker will face several important misconceptions about pain that must be addressed with the patient and family to assure rapid, successful control of the symptom. The most common misconceptions are listed in Table 8–1. It is important to understand the differences between acute and cancer-associated chronic pain. Cancer-associated chronic pain is not associated with changes in vital signs as noted in acute pain. These signs are mediated by the autonomic nervous system to which chronic pain has adapted, and the classic sweating, anxiety, and facies are no longer present. Thus, the individual with chronic pain may develop many adaptive coping mechanisms, which mask the "characteristic" findings seen in people with acute pain. These can assume many different forms (e.g., humor, distraction by conversation, music, art, writing, or watching television). Thus, the person with chronic cancer-associated pain may not "look like they are having pain." The health care worker, who is caring for these patients must allow the patient to quantitate their own individual pain.

TABLE 8–1    Common Misconceptions about Cancer-Associated Pain

All cancer is painful.

The amount of pain is related to the extent of the cancer.

Strong pain medicines cause addiction.

Taking pain medicine too early will interfere with it working "when you really need it."

People who complain are not good patients.

## ❖ Assessment of Pain

A comprehensive assessment is the foundation for constructing the treatment plan. Since pain is subjective, the patient's responses are integral to the plan. Table 8–2 outlines a series of questions to ask individuals regarding their pain. The initial pain assessment may be more comprehensive than the ongoing assessments. It is helpful for the health care worker to use a pain flow sheet to document and evaluate the interventions used to manage the person's pain. It is also helpful for the patient to keep a pain diary to document the pain experience as it is happening. An example of a flow sheet and pain diary are found in Appendix II.

Never assume that a laughing patient is free of pain. One still needs to use the appropriate tools to ask the patient about their pain level. Patient/family education regarding the pain in terms they are able to understand is imperative to good pain management. The goal is to involve patients in their individual treatment plan.

## ❖ Management of Pain

Several principles are important to consider when managing pain in the hospice setting. These are listed in Table 8–3. The clinician must initially decide if pharmacologic, nonpharmacologic, or a combination of both are to be introduced.

TABLE 8–2  Components of a Comprehensive Pain Assessment

Ask the individual:

1. To characterize the pain by location, intensity, duration and quality. Use a pain assessment tool. See Appendix I.

   Location: Ask the patient to point to the area of pain and to describe whether or not the pain radiates to another part of the body.
   Quality: Ask the patient to describe how the pain feels (e.g., burning, aching, throbbing).
   Intensity: Use a pain intensity scale. See Appendix I.
   Duration: Ask the patient to describe the pain as constant or intermittent.

2. To describe aggravating and relieving factors (e.g., what makes your pain better? What makes your pain worse?).

3. To describe how the pain interferes with activities of daily living.

4. To describe the impact on his/her psychosocial state (e.g., meaning of the pain, past experiences with pain, concerns about using opioids, changes in mood).

5. To describe responses to previous pharmacologic and nonpharmacologic interventions.

6. To keep a diary that includes all of the above issues. See Appendix II.

Source: Jacox, A. K., et al. *Management of Cancer Pain.* Agency for Health Care Policy and Research, 1994.

TABLE 8–3    Principles of Pain Relief in Hospice Care

1. Whenever possible, give medication by mouth. Oral medication is the most convenient and cost effective.

2. Medication should be given by the clock depending on the pharmacokinetics of the drug being used. Additional doses of the drug should be prescribed for "breakthrough" (i.e., pain that occurs before the next scheduled dose).

3. Use the World Health Organization's Pain Treatment Ladder as a guide for the type of drug to be used for the amount of pain that the person is experiencing.

4. Tailor the treatment plan to the individual's needs.

5. Review the regimen and its pain relief often.

Source: Jacox, A. K., et al. Management of Cancer Pain. Agency for Health Care Policy and Research, 1994.

## Nonpharmacologic Approaches

Although pharmacologic treatment may be the most common form of pain management, many nonpharmacologic techniques have proven to be effective in the relief of pain.[13] Many of these techniques will have been used by the patient even prior to being seen. Remember to ask the patient about them during the initial assessment. Most of these techniques can be taught and applied by family, friends, or significant others in the patient's life. The application of some of these techniques allows them an opportunity to "do something" for their loved one. Nonpharmacologic treatments are usually divided into physical and psychosocial modalities. Physical modalities include cutaneous stimulation—i.e., massage, thermal manipulation, vibration, pressure, exercises, immobilization, transcutaneous electrical nerve stimulation (TENS), and acupuncture.[14] Psychosocial modalities include relaxation and imagery, distraction and reframing, education, psychotherapy, support groups, and pastoral counseling.

### Cutaneous Stimulation

These techniques are suggested for pain associated with muscle tension or spasm. Cutaneous stimulation often distracts the patient from the pain and may enhance relaxation and decrease anxiety.[15] Appropriate exercise is dependent on the patient's physical stamina. Active range of motion and participation in daily activities may also enhance the patient's feeling of well being. Exercise should be limited to self-administered range of motion during periods of acute exacerbation of pain.[16] Immobilization may be used during periods of acute pain (e.g., stabilize a fracture due to bone metastasis). Counterstimulation techniques include TENS and acupuncture. TENS uses low-voltage electricity to relieve pain. Acupuncture is believed to correct imbalances of energy in the body by inserting special needles into specific body points.[17] TENS and acupuncture should only be used by specially-trained health care professionals.

## Psychosocial Interventions

Psychosocial interventions may include cognitive techniques which are designed to influence how the patient interprets pain through events and bodily sensations. They may also include behavioral techniques that assist patients in developing appropriate skills to cope with pain.[18] Relaxation and imagery are designed to promote mental relaxation by decreasing anxiety, and physical relaxation by reducing skeletal muscle tension. Some examples include progressive muscle relaxation, meditation, and slow, rhythmic breathing. Imagery may be used as a form of distraction from pain, to produce relaxation, or to produce an image of pain relief. Distraction comes in many forms. Here the hospice volunteer, as a visitor, may play an important and unique role. Music and art have also been found to be effective in managing pain. Music can be used with relaxation and visual imagery or can serve as a form of distraction. The roles of music and art therapists are described in more detail in Chapter 5. The results of two studies have suggested that distraction, position change, massage, and heat were useful in controlling pain.[19] Psychosocial interventions may include cognitive techniques that are designed to influence how the patient interprets pain through events and bodily sensations. They may also include behavioral techniques which assist patients in developing appropriate skills to cope with pain.

## *Pharmacologic Approaches*

When confronted with a patient in pain, the clinician completes the assessment and usually begins therapy with medication. Again, in hospice work, nonpharmacologic techniques alone or in combination might be important to consider even initially. This is particularly important in an elderly person with multisystem disease receiving many other medications or in a person where drug administration may be problematic. The most commonly employed medications, dose, frequency of administration, formulation, and route of delivery are listed in Tables 8–4 through 8–7. The costs associated with the treatment of pain have been reported in detail elsewhere.[20,21] The oral route of administration is preferred because it is the most convenient and cost effective method of administration. The intramuscular route should be avoided because it is painful, especially in a debilitated person.

## *Selection of Medication(s) for Pain Management*

Three major classes of drugs are used alone, in combination, or sequentially to decrease the magnitude of the patient's pain. The three broad groupings are:

1. Nonsteroidal anti-inflammatory drugs (NSAIDS), including acetaminophen.
2. Agonist, antagonist, and mixed agonist-antagonist opioids.

TABLE 8–4    Acetaminophen and NSAIDS—
Usual Dose for Adults and Children ≥ 50kg Body Weight

| Drug | Dose |
| --- | --- |
| Acetaminophen | 650mg q4h<br>975mg q6h |
| Aspirin | 650mg q4h<br>975mg q6h |
| Ibuprofen | 400–600mg q6h |
| Choline magnesium trisalicylate | 1,000–1,500mg tid |
| Naproxen | 250–275mg q6–8h |
| Sodium salicylate | 325–650mg q3–4h |
| Salsate | 750mg qid |

*Sources:* Jacox, A. K., et al. *Management of Cancer Pain.* Agency for Health Care Policy and Research, 1994.

Watt-Watson, J. H., and Donovan, M. I., eds. *Pain Management: Nursing Perspective.* St. Louis: Mosby–Year Book, 1992.

TABLE 8–5    Opioid Analgesics—Approximate Equianalgesic Dose

Dose Equivalent in Opioid-Naive Adults and Children ≥ 50 kg Body Weight

| Drug | Oral | Parenteral |
| --- | --- | --- |
| Morphine | 30mg q3–4h | 10mg q3–4h |
| Morphine, controlled release | 90–120mg q12h | N/A |
| Hydromorphone | 7.5mg q3–4h | 1.5mg q3–4h |
| Methadone | 20mg q6–8h | 10mg q6–8h |
| Oxycodone | 30mg q3–4h | N/A |
| Codeine | 180–200mg q3–4h | 130mg q3–4h |

*Source:* Jacox, A. K., et al. *Management of Cancer Pain.* Agency for Health Care Policy and Research, 1994.

3. Adjuvant analgesics. This is a broad group of drugs that acts alone as analgesics or synergistic to one of the above classes of analgesics. These agents span a broad spectrum of drugs ranging from anticonvulsants to antidepressants, to those with specific inhibitory function as inhibitors of excitatory amino acids in the nervous system. The following is a very brief review of these agents. The reader is referred to the many excellent textbooks on treating pain for greater detail.[22,23]

## Nonsteroidal Anti-Inflammatory Drugs (NSAIDS)

Nonsteroidal anti-inflammatory drugs (NSAIDS), which are quite numerous, are employed for a variety of pain syndromes. In particular,

TABLE 8–6    Adjuvant Analgesics

| Drug | Approximate Adult Daily Dose Range (Oral) |
|---|---|
| *Corticosteroids* | |
| Dexamethasone | 16–96 mg (also IV/SC) |
| Prednisone | 40–100mg |
| *Antidepressants* | |
| Amitriptyline | 10–150mg |
| Nortriptyline | 10–150mg |
| Doxepin | 10–150mg |
| Imipramine | 10–150mg |
| *Anticonvulsants* | |
| Carbamazepine | 200–1,600mg |
| Phenytoin | 300–500mg |
| *Local anesthetics/antiarrythmics* | |
| Mexiletine | 450–600mg |
| Lidocaine | 5mg/kg (also IV/SC) |
| Tocainide | 20mg/kg |

*Sources:* Jacox, A. K., et al. *Management of Cancer Pain.* Agency for Health Care Policy and Research, 1994.

Kaye, P. *Notes on Symptom Control in Hospice and Palliative Care.* Essex, CT: Hospice Education Institute, 1990.

these agents are used for mild to moderate nociceptive pain and pain associated with inflammation. They are especially useful in relieving the pain associated with bony metastasis. In the World Health Organization's (WHO) pain treatment ladder, these agents form the first rung. In addition to their known toxicity related to gastrointestinal bleeding and renal failure, several specific problems must be kept in mind during their administration. First, they are subject to the "ceiling effect" in their analgesic efficacy. This effect is seen when a drug no longer will produce pain relief above a certain dosage. Second, there are unique toxicity in special populations (e.g., delirium in the elderly). Third, there is no data that one class of NSAID is more efficacious than another or that one is less toxic. The use of the nonacelated salicylates might be a better choice in a patient with general bleeding tendencies, as these agents are less likely to produce platelet dysfunction. Otherwise, cost is a good guide in selection.

## Opioids

In choosing an opioid the WHO suggests beginning with an opioid such as codeine or oxycodone. Adding the opioid to the NSAID should occur within a few days of initiating pain therapy to bring the pain under control as quickly as possible. The opioid dose should be escalated quickly. If the pain is not under control as the patient perceives it, within a few days the clinician should convert to a strong opioid such as morphine,

TABLE 8–7    Opioids, NSAIDS and Adjuvant Analgesics

| Drug | Formulation |
| --- | --- |
| Morphine | tablet liquid parenteral |
| Morphine, controlled release | tablet |
| Hydromorphone | tablet suppository parenteral |
| Methadone | tablet parenteral |
| Oxycodone | tablet liquid |
| Codeine | tablet parenternal |
| Acetaminophen | tablet liquid suppository |
| Aspirin | tablet liquid suppository |
| Ibuprofen | tablet liquid |
| Choline magnesium trisalicylate | tablet liquid |
| Naproxen | tablet |
| Sodium salicylate | tablet |
| Salsate | tablet |
| Dexamethasone | tablet parenteral |
| Prednisone | tablet |
| Amitriptyline | tablet |
| Nortriptyline | tablet |
| Doxepin | tablet |
| Imiprimine | tablet |
| Mexiletine | tablet |
| Lidocaine | parenteral |
| Tocainide | tablet |

hydromorphone, or in selected situations, fentanyl. Table 8–5 gives the relative conversion factors for these opioids. Pain should be controlled with an immediate release preparation before changing to a sustained release opioid. Note that the antagonists and mixed agonist-antagonists are not included. They are not used because of the adverse interactions with the pure agonists. Also, as suggested above, if the pain is not being controlled easily with "weak" opioids, convert early to the "strong" opioid. Meperidine, although it is an agonist opioid, is not recommended for chronic pain. Its toxic metabolite, normeperidine, accumulates with repetitive dosing, which may lead to central nervous system toxicity in the form of tremors, confusion, and seizures. Although it is relatively inexpensive, methadone also has a metabolite with a very long half life that produces somnolence, making it a difficult agent to use.[24] A major advantage of several of the strong opioids is they can be given by a variety of routes of administration. The sublingual route has been suggested for morphine, although controlled clinical trials are lacking.[25]

## Adjuvant Analgesics for Cancer-Associated Pain

Adjuvant drugs are used to enhance the analgesic effects of the other analgesics, but the term *adjuvant* also applies to their ability to enhance the analgesic properties of the opioids (e.g., dexamethasone or a muscle relaxant added to morphine). However, adjuvant analgesics are mainly used in patients with two or more types of pain (e.g., bone pain and neuropathic pain in the same individual), to provide analgesia for specific types of pain (e.g., neuropathic), or to provide specific analgesia (e.g., capsaicin in diabetic neuropathy).[26] Headache due to increased intracranial pressure is a common result of intracerebral metastasis and is most effectively treated with dexamethasone and radiation therapy. Table 8–6 lists the commonly employed adjuvant analgesics. References for these agents are as indicated.[27–30]

## Miscellaneous Medications

A variety of medications and techniques have very specific indications in relieving cancer-associated pain. Radiation therapy can be used in the treatment of bone pain, nerve compression by cancer, bone metastasis, and in the relief of headache caused by metastatic or primary cancer in the brain. A new agent, Strontium 89, a radiopharmaceutical, has recently been shown to be at least partially effective in treating bony metastatic sites, particularly when the clinician is faced with multiple painful areas.[31] Finally, both neurosurgical and anesthetic techniques are available to treat pain. The reader is referred to the article by Hankin and Justins for more details about these special interventions.[32]

## ❖ Summary

Pain is often a part of the clinical problem the clinician must treat in the person with cancer. Since this symptom can lead to terrible suffering with a loss of quality of life, every hospice professional must be an expert in its relief. Factors that are critical to this mission are:

1. Make certain that you have allowed the person, particularly children and the elderly, to express pain.
2. A variety of tools are available to measure the pain the individual is experiencing. Choose the most effective tools for the person you are evaluating.
3. Once pain is assessed, multiple interventions are available that can be utilized. Most are easily mastered and must be part of the armamentarium of the hospice professional.
4. The doses recommended by various authors are to be used as general guidelines and modified for the individual patient.
5. On occasion, even the experts are challenged. In these circumstances, consultation with other professionals might be the best choice to relieve the person's pain. The compassionate, competent hospice professional will not hesitate to seek such advice.

## ❖ References

1. Foley, K.M. "The Treatment of Cancer Pain." *New England Journal of Medicine, 313*:84–95, 1985.
2. McGuire, D.B. "Comprehensive and Multidimensional Assessment and Measurement of Pain." *Journal of Pain and Symptom Management, 7*:312–319, 1992.
3. World Health Organization. *Cancer Pain Relief.* Geneva: World Health Organization, 1986.
4. National Hospice Organization. *Standards of a Hospice Program of Care.* Arlington, VA: National Hospice Organization, 1993.
5. Jacox, A.K., et al. *Management of Cancer Pain.* Rockville, MD: Agency for Health Care Policy and Research, 1994.
6. Spross, J.A., McGuire, D.B., and Schmitt, R.M. Oncology Nursing Society Position Paper on Cancer Pain. "Part I. Introduction, Scope of Nursing Practice Regarding Cancer Pain, Ethics & Practice." *Oncology Nursing Forum, 17*(4):595–614, 1990.
7. Spross, J.A., McGuire, D.B., and Schmitt, R.M. Oncology Nursing Society Position Paper on Cancer Pain. "Part II. Education & Research, Cancer Pain Management Resources." *Oncology Nursing Forum, 17*(5):751–760, 1990.
8. Spross, J.A., McGuire, D.B., and Schmitt, R.M. Oncology Nursing Society Position Paper on Cancer Pain. "Part III. Nursing Administration, Social Policy, Pediatric Cancer Pain, Appendices." *Oncology Nursing Forum, 17*(6):943–955, 1990.
9. American Pain Society. *Principles of Analgesic Use in the Treatment of Acute Pain and Cancer Pain,* 3rd ed. Skokie, IL: American Pain Society, 1992.
10. Weissman, D.E., Burchman, S.L., Dinndorf, P.A., and Dahl, J.L., eds. *Handbook of Cancer Pain Management,* 3rd ed. Wisconsin Pain Initiative, 1992.
11. Chapman, C.R., and Bonica, J.J., eds. *Cancer Pain.* Kalamazoo: The Upjohn Co., 1992.
12. Foley, K. "Cancer Pain Syndromes." *Journal of Pain and Symptom Management, 2*(2):13–17, 1986.

13. Foley, K. "The Treatment of Cancer Pain." *New England Journal of Medicine,* 313:84–95, 1985.
14. Barbour, L.A., McGuire, D.B., and Kirchhoff, K.T. "Nonanalgesic Methods of Pain Control Used by Cancer Outpatients," *Oncology Nursing Forum,* 13:56–60, 1986.
15. McCaffery, M., and Bebe, A. *Pain: Clinical Manual for Nursing Practice.* St. Louis: C.V. Mosby, 1989.
16. Lee, M.H.M., Itoh, M., Yang, G.W., and Eason, A.L. "Physical Therapy and Rehabilitation Medicine." In J.J. Bonica, ed. *The Management of Pain,* 2nd ed., vol. 2. Philadelphia: Lea & Febiger, 1990.
17. Rankin-Box, D.F., ed. *Complementary Health Therapies: A Guide for Nurses and the Caring Professions.* London: Chapman & Hall, 1980.
18. Doyle, D., Hanks, G.W.C., and MacDonald, N. eds. *Oxford Textbook of Palliative Medicine.* Oxford: Oxford University Press, 1993.
19. Donovan, M.I. "Nursing Assessment of Cancer Pain." *Seminaries in Oncology Nursing,* 1:109–115, 1985.
20. Ferrell, B.R., and Griffith, H. "Cost Issues Related to Pain Management: Report from the Cancer Pain Panel of the Agency for Health Care Policy and Research." *Journal of Pain and Symptom Management,* 9(4):221–234, 1994.
21. Kolassa, M. "Guidance for Clinicians in Discerning and Comparing the Price of Pharmaceutical Agents." *Journal of Pain and Symptom Management,* 9(4):235–243, 1994.
22. Johanson, G. *Physician's Handbook of Symptom Relief in Terminal Care,* 4th ed. Santa Rosa, CA: Sonoma County Academic Foundation for Excellence in Medicine, 1993.
23. Kaye, P. *Notes on Symptom Control in Hospice and Palliative Care.* Essex, CT: Hospice Education Institute, 1990.
24. Enck, R.E. *The Medical Care of Terminally Ill Patients.* Baltimore: John Hopkins University Press, 1994.
25. Pitorak, E.F., and Kraus, J.C. "Pain Control with Sublingual Morphine." *The American Journal of Hospice Care,* March/April (1987):39–41.
26. Watson, C.P.N. "Topical Capsaicin as an Adjuvant Analgesic." *Journal of Pain and Symptom Management,* 9:425–433, 1994.
27. Watson, C.P.N. "Antidepressant Drugs as Adjuvant Analgesics." *Journal of Pain and Symptom Management,* 9:393–405, 1994.
28. Waldman, H.J. "Centrally Acting Skeletal Muscle Relaxants and Associated Drugs." *J Pain Symp Manage,* 9:434–441, 1994.
29. Watanabe, S., and Bruero, E. "Corticosteroids as Adjuvant Analgesics." *Journal of Pain and Symptom Management,* 9:442–445, 1994.
30. Patt, R.B., Proper, G., and Reddy, S. "The Neuroleptics as Adjuvant Analgesics." *Journal of Pain and Symptom Management,* 9:446–453, 1994.
31. Kovner, F., Ron, I.G., Levita, M., and Chaitchik, S. "Strontium 89 Therapy in a Patient with Carcinoma of Unknown Origin and Incurable Pain from Bone Metastases." *Journal of Pain and Symptom Management,* 8:47–51, 1993.
32. Hanks, G.W., and Justins, D.M. "Cancer Pain: Management." *Lancet,* 339:1031–1036, 1992.

## ❖ For Further Reading

Bruera, E. "Issues of Symptom Control in Patients with Advanced Cancer." *American Journal of Hospice Palliative Care*, March/April (1993):12–18.

Bruero, E., et al. "A Prospective Multicenter Assessment of the Edmonton Staging System for Cancer Pain." *Journal of Pain and Symptom Management*, 10(5):348–355, 1995.

Buchholz, W.M. "Terminal Care, Part 2: Treating the Whole Person." *Journal of the American Academy of Physicians' Assistants*, 6:203–209, 1993.

Burchman, S.L., and Pagel, P.S. "Implementation of a Formal Treatment Agreement for Outpatient Management of Chronic Nonmalignant Pain with Opioid Analgesics." *Journal of Pain and Symptom Management*, 10(7):556–563, 1995.

de Stoutz, N.D., and Suarez-Almazor, M. "Opioid Rotation for Toxicity Reduction in Terminal Cancer Patients." *Journal of Pain and Symptom Management*, 10(5):378–384, 1995.

Ernst, E.E., and Fialka, V. "Ice Freezes Pain? A Review of the Clinical Effectiveness of Analgesic Cold Therapy." *Journal of Pain and Symptom Management*, 9(1):56–59, 1994.

Ferrell, B.R., McCaffery, M., and Grant, M. "Clinical Decision Making and Pain." *Cancer Nursing*, 14(6):289–297, 1991.

Ferrell-Torry, A.T., and Glick, O.J. "The Use of Therapeutic Massage as a Nursing Intervention to Modify Anxiety and the Perception of Cancer Pain." *Cancer Nursing*, 16(2):93–101, 1992.

Fromm, G.H. "Baclofen as an Adjuvant Analgesic." *Journal of Pain and Symptom Management*, 9(8):500–509, 1994.

Kan, M.K. "Palliation of Bone Pain in Patients with Metastatic Cancer Using Strontium-89 (Metastron)." *Cancer Nursing*, 18(4):286–291, 1995.

Levy, M.H. "Pharmacologic Management of Cancer Pain." *Seminars in Oncology*, 21(6):718–739, 1994.

McCorquodale, S., DeFaye, B., and Bruera, E. "Pain Control in an Alcoholic Cancer Patient." *Journal of Pain and Symptom Management*, 8(3):177–180, 1993.

McGuire, D.B., Yarbro, C.H., and Ferrell, B.R., eds. *Cancer Pain Management*, 2nd ed. Boston: Jones and Bartlett, 1995.

Mignault, G.G. et al. "Control of Cancer-Related Pain with MS Contin: A Comparison Between 12-Hourly and 8-Hourly Administration." *Journal of Pain and Symptom Management*, 10(6):416–422, 1995.

Reddy, S., and Patt, R.B. "The Benzodiazepines as Adjuvant Analgesics." *Journal of Pain and Symptom Management*, 9(8):510–514, 1994.

Watt-Watson, J.H., and Donovan, M.I., eds. *Pain Management: Nursing Perspective*. St. Louis: Mosby–Year Book, 1992.

Weinrich, S.P., and Weinrich, M.C. "The Effect of Massage on Pain in Cancer Patients." *Applied Nursing Research*, 3(4):140–145, 1990.

Wesson, D.R., Ling, W., and Smith, D.E. "Prescription of Opioids for Treatment of Pain in Patients with Addictive Disease." *Journal of Pain and Symptom Management*, 8(5):289–296, 1993.

Zenz, M., Donner, B., and Strumpf, M. "Withdrawal Symptoms during Therapy with Transdermal Fentanyl?" *Journal of Pain and Symptom Management*, 9(1):54–55, 1994.

# ❖ Chapter 9

# Symptom Management

WALTER B. FORMAN

DENICE C. SHEEHAN

Pain is an obvious symptom that must be controlled in the terminally ill person. The previous chapter reviews this issue and gives the reader a comprehensive bibliography. But what is known about other symptoms that the person with a terminal illness may face? Actually, we know quite a lot, particularly in regard to their frequency and accompanying manifestations. In a recent review of 1,635 patients entering a pain clinic, Grond and colleagues found that 94 percent of the patients reported symptoms other than pain.[1] Of this population, 80 percent reported more than one symptom and 15 percent reported more than five symptoms with an average of three symptoms per patient. These included insomnia (59 percent), anorexia (48 percent), constipation (33 percent), sweating (28 percent), nausea (27 percent), dyspnea (24 percent), dysphagia (20 percent), neuropsychiatric symptoms (20 percent), vomiting (20 percent), urinary symptoms (14 percent), dyspepsia (11 percent), paresis (10 percent), diarrhea (6 percent), pruritus (6 percent), and dermatological symptoms (3 percent). They were also able to relate the symptom(s) to the site of the cancer with the highest number of symptoms being in patients with cancer of the respiratory system. Of even more interest, gender, age, and tumor stage were not correlated with the type and number of symptoms.

In light of this information, a few general comments are in order. In the hustle and bustle of today's health care system it is important to listen to the patient. They can have more than one symptom that needs attention. Pay particular attention to the list of medications that are being taken including over-the-counter medications, homeopathic herbs, and so forth. When you feel comfortable that you have all the problems in hand, the physical examination should complement your historical facts. Now for the hard part—what medications to institute. We suggest that you keep it as simple as possible. A good target is to attempt to keep the list to five or fewer medications. For example, in a person with nausea, anorexia, pain, and insomnia, the combination of morphine for the pain, dexamethasone for the nausea and anorexia, and haloperidol to assist in controlling the nausea and insomnia might be a simple but effective regimen.

## ❖ Respiratory

Dyspnea is the subjective sensation of difficulty in breathing. It is not necessarily related to exertion. Dyspnea compels the individual to increase ventilation or reduce activity.[2] As with pain, the individual is the only one who can accurately judge the presence and severity of dyspnea. It may be caused by muscle weakness due to cancer; primary disease of muscle as in amyotrophic lateral sclerosis (ALS); abnormal diaphragm or chest wall function secondary to physical interference or neurologic innervation as in pleural effusion; obstructive lung diseases; and chemotherapy-induced neuropathies. Other causes include primary disease of the lung tissue, as in fibrosis due to radiation therapy or chemotherapy with bleomycin or alkylators. Underlying disease may result from tobacco abuse. Dyspnea may also be caused by diseases that cause abnormal blood flow through the lungs, as in heart failure and pulmonary embolism. Finally, psychosocial components causing anxiety may also be associated with the sensation of dyspnea.

The fear associated with dyspnea often centers around the distress related to the sensation of suffocating or smothering. Reassurance and prompt relief of the symptom is essential for relieving this manifestation. Treatment is directed at the underlying cause. However, opioids relieve dyspnea resulting from many different etiologies. They have been shown to be effective in relieving dyspnea due to cancer[3] as well as chronic obstructive lung disease.[4] If the patient is not currently taking an opioid, morphine sulfate 2.5–5mg p.o. every four hours is an appropriate place to begin.[5,6] In patients currently taking an opioid for pain, Twycross and Lack recommend increasing the dose by 50 percent.[6] Storey recommends increasing the dose by 30–50 percent every twelve to twenty-four hours until the patient is comfortable or develops unacceptable side effects.[7] Bruera and colleagues suggest 2.5 times the patient's regular dose for pain to overcome tolerance.[3] They noted a shorter duration for morphine's effect on dyspnea when compared to the analgesic effect. Therefore, time and dose should be adjusted according to the individual patient's needs. Nebulized morphine has also been shown to be effective in the treatment of dyspnea in patients with end-stage chronic lung disease and heart failure.[8] Corticosteroids are used to reduce inflammation and edema around the tumor. They are effective in treating dyspnea related to tracheal and bronchial obstruction as well as superior vena cava syndrome and lymphangitis carcinomatosis. The recommended dose of dexamethasone ranges from 4–16mg p.o. daily.[2,5,9] Benzodiazapines such as lorazepam have also been reported to be effective in treating dyspnea with an anxiety component. Doses range from 1–2mg p.o. every four to six hours when the patient is also receiving an opioid. Lorazepam has a short half life and does not have active metabolites that might interfere with treatment goals.[6–9] Chlorpromazine has been recommended as another alternative to control dyspnea in dying cancer patients.[10]

Many effective nonpharmacologic interventions are available for the treatment of dyspnea. A bedside fan or open window can provide a cool breeze. The air should be directed towards the patient's face.[5,6,11,12] Cool cloths on the face are also very helpful. Positioning techniques include elevating the head of the bed and encouraging the patient to sit on the edge of the bed or chair and to lean forward supporting the arms and upper body on a table. Pursed-lip breathing or deep breathing are other options. The use of supplemental oxygen was found to decrease the intensity of dyspnea in terminally ill cancer patients who were hypoxic and experienced dyspnea at rest.[4] Relaxation therapy has been shown to be very effective in reducing dyspnea, anxiety, and airway obstruction in patients with chronic obstructive pulmonary disease.[13] An individual who stays with the patient to provide a calming presence may also be extremely helpful.[5,6,11]

## Cough

The incidence of cough in terminally ill cancer patients has been estimated at 50 percent. This number increases to 80 percent in those with bronchogenic cancer.[6] A wet cough is productive when the patient is able to cough effectively. It may be caused by infection, heart failure, or mechanical irritation due to cancer. This same wet cough may be nonproductive if the patient is unable to cough effectively due to weakness or fatigue. A dry, nonproductive cough may be caused by pulmonary fibrosis, bronchospasm, pleural effusion, or mechanical irritation due to cancer. Bronchial irritation related to smoking may also contribute to the cough.

A persistent cough is not only distressing to the patient and family members, but can lead to serious complications. For example, cough syncope occurs when a fall in systolic blood pressure leads to loss of consciousness. Increase venous pressure during coughing episodes may cause headache, retinal, conjunctival, or intracranial hemorrhage. Patients with bony metastases or multiple myeloma are at higher risk for pathological fractures of the ribs. Chronic cough often leads to pain in the chest and ribs as well as physical exhaustion.[14]

The goal of therapy is to attempt to uncover the cause of the cough and then apply appropriate therapy. Infections may be treated with appropriate antibiotics. Persistent bronchospasm may be alleviated by using bronchodilators and corticosteroids. Pulmonary metastases and lymphangitis carcinomatosis are treated with corticosteroids.[6,14] If pleural effusions are drained, it is important to include a sclerosing agent to prevent another effusion. It is interesting to note that it takes two to four weeks to obtain significant antitussive benefits following the cessation of smoking. Mucolytic agents are helpful in decreasing the viscosity of bronchial secretions. A humidifier placed at the foot of the bed or nebulized saline may be very effective.[6] Antihistamines and anticholinergic medications may be helpful in reducing respiratory secretions. However, care must be taken to prevent increasing sputum viscosity. A dry cough is often suppressed with antitussive medications such as codeine and morphine. The recommended dose for codeine is 8–30mg p.o. every four hours. Morphine sulfate 5–20mg p.o. is given every four hours. The antitussive dose is usually less than the analgesic dose.[14] There seems to be some controversy regarding commercially available cough syrups. Those containing hycosine or codeine may be beneficial. However, some experts believe that the liquid carrier for the active agents is the most important component because it reduces pharyngeal sensitivity.[2,6,14]

## Noisy Respirations

Many patients experience noisy respirations during the final hours prior to death. Oral and pulmonary secretions collect in the pharynx and the patient is unable to cough to clear the trachea. The sound is more distressing to friends and family than to the patient who is usually unconscious. Repositioning may be all that is necessary to stop the noisy respirations. Those visiting the patient need to be reassured that this change in respiratory sounds does not mean the patient is suffering or is uncomfortable. Anticholinergic medications suppress the production of secretions and may sometimes produce paradoxical excitation especially after repeated doses. Atropine 0.4–0.8mg may be given subcutaneously every two to four hours. Scopolamine 0.3–0.8mg may be administered subcutaneously every two to four hours or a scopolamine patch may be applied every seventy-two hours.[11,14] Scopolamine 0.8–3.2mg/day may be given by continuous subcutaneous infusion. Ditropan 5–10mg three times per day is another alternative to dry secretions.[7] Suction is rarely helpful and may cause more secretions and discomfort. Those patients who are slightly dehydrated have less secretions. Therefore, they are less likely to experience noisy respirations.

## ❖ Gastrointestinal

Gastrointestinal complaints are both numerous and multifactorial in the hospice setting. Thus, the practitioner must be able to distinguish nausea due to increased intracranial pressure versus that observed in gastric paresis caused by opioids, diarrhea secondary to antibiotic therapy, and that due to constipation. Of course some of the same symptoms can be caused by two or more synergistic mechanisms. In this brief introduction to common gastrointestinal symptoms in palliative care, the most commonly diagnosed disorders and their treatment will be considered.

## Anorexia/Nausea/Emesis

The loss of the desire to eat is one of the more distressing symptoms to both the family and the patient. It can also herald the onset of the most difficult to treat syndromes in palliative care—the cancer anorexia cachexia syndrome. The most overlooked causes of anorexia are diseases of the oral cavity. Maintaining oral hygiene is critical to allow adequate oral intake. Problems can be primarily due to dental abnormalities (e.g., caries, poorly fitting appliances, infection), or secondarily due to damage from radiation, chemotherapy, or surgery. Oral fungal infections can also affect the esophagus causing dysphagia and loss of appetite. Other etiologies of these symptoms include, but are not limited to, obstruction of the upper gastrointestinal tract, abnormal tastes and/or smells, and inflammatory states such as ulcer disease. Central etiologies include central nervous system disorders such as metastasis, delirium, drugs, and the central effect of various metabolic disorders (e.g., hypercalcemia, azotemia, and systemic illnesses). Finally, patients with advanced malignancies can develop a syndrome of anorexia, weakness, easy fatigue, nausea, and emesis. This malady, known as the cancer anorexia cachexia syndrome, is probably due to kinin generation by the interaction of the particular malignancy and the inflammatory system. The biochemical abnormality is the production of an excessive amount of lactic acid from carbohydrate metabolism, which is thought to be the putative agent in the etiology of the syndrome.[15] Treatment is initially directed at mouth care and requires an adequate and accurate assessment. Is the patient noting xerostomia (dry mouth) related to decreased saliva formation from therapy or from other causes? Table 9–1 is a simplified approach to mouth care modified from Regnard.[16]

The cachexia caused by anorexia can be approached by several techniques. However, there is no satisfactory regimen at present to relieve this situation. It is important to explain to the patient and family why the individual is unable to eat, what you can and cannot do to reverse the situation, and the psychosocial role of food in the care of the terminally ill person. It is important to note the difference between starving to death from lack of food, which is remediable by providing adequate intake, and the situation in cancer cachexia in which food, no matter what form or amount, cannot overcome the metabolic defect. The professional caregiver can assist in the following areas. Oral nutrition, despite its limitations in terms of calories delivered per unit time and volume, remains the simplest, most ideal treatment, and is associated with the least morbidity and mortality of any other route of delivering calories and fluids. In the terminally ill, the use of other forms of nutrition is controversial at best.

How should one deliver oral intake to a terminally ill patient? Remember that comfort—not calories—is what is important. Therefore, patients should be extended the opportunity to choose the food(s) of their choice, the time that it will be eaten, the quantity to be eaten, and where the activity is to take place. Be certain that the family and other caregivers are comfortable with the goals, otherwise the appearance of the patient and their physical deterioration will be extremely disconcerting to all. The agents used to stimulate appetite include corticosteroids, progestational agents such as megesterol acetate, cannabinoids, and a variety of other drugs such as hydrazine

TABLE 9–1    Mouth Care in Hospice and Palliative Care

| Problem | Findings | Etiology | Treatment |
|---------|----------|----------|-----------|
| Maintenance | ——— | ——— | Vigorous hygiene (brushing, flossing, alcohol free rinses). Dental consultation if at high risk |
| Dry mouth | Poor salivary flow; viscous secretions | Radiation, drugs, dehydration $O_2$ | Hygiene, artificial saliva, pilocarpine, change medication, ice chips, gum or hard candy |
| Painful mouth | Red, fissured tongue | Dentures, infection | See above. Also protective mixtures (sulcrafate solution), diphenhydramine; magnesium hydroxide; viscous xylocaine |
| Infected mouth | White plaques, ulcerations, purulent discharge | Fungal or viral infection, malignancy | Specific Rx, topical analgesia |

Source: Regnard, C., and Fitton, S. "Mouth Care: A Flow Diagram." Palliative Medicine, 3:67–69, 1989.

sulfate and cyproheptadine. Several trials have suggested that in AIDS patients the cannaboids might be effective,[11] while hydrazine sulfate was not effective in patients with advanced colorectal cancer in regards to quality of life and weight gain.[17] Clinical data suggest hydrazine sulfate might be efficacious in improving the nutritional status and median survival in patients with non-small cell lung cancer.[18] However, a randomized trial did not confirm these findings.[19] The author favors the use of dexamethasone 4mg qam for those individuals where "something must be given." A feeling of well being is often achieved with corticosteroids thereby increasing appetite.

## Intestinal Obstruction

Once patients have failed surgical relief or are so ill that surgery would increase mortality and not quality of life, nonsurgical options must be considered. In the past, patients have been left with the unhappy prospect

TABLE 9-2   Drug Regimen for Organic Intestinal Obstruction

---

Opioid to lessen any colicky pain

Steroid to decrease the edema

Antiemetic to control the nausea and vomiting

Octreotide to decrease secretions

---

Source: Ripamonti, C. "Management of Bowel Obstruction in Advanced Cancer Patients." Journal of Pain and Symptom Management, 9:193–200, 1994.

of being attached to an intravenous line and nasogastric suction for the remainder of their lives. With the addition of octreotide, a somatostatin analog that decreases gastrointestinal secretions, the palliative care worker can substantially improve the quality of life by obviating the need for nasogastric suction and intravenous fluids. In the person with intestinal obstruction, the regimen should include an opioid to lessen colicky pain, a steroid to decrease the peritumor edema, and an antiemetic such as haloperidol and octreotide. These drugs can be given subcutaneously as a continuous infusion or the octreotide can be given as twice daily injections. This regimen is outlined in Table 9-2. In the appropriate clinical setting, the initial consideration should be to rule out gastric stasis from opioid therapy. A course of metoclopromide (10mg t.i.d. orally if tolerated) or by continuous subcutaneous infusion (60–90mg/24hrs q.s. 100ml 5% D/W) over 24hrs should lessen the emesis.[6,14,16,20,21]

## Constipation

The individual who has dry, cracked stools that over 25 percent of the time require straining in order to pass is constipated. Stool frequency is only important in regard to how it has changed for the particular person. The average person has five to seven stools per week. Therapy is directed at:

1. Diet: Many patients are unable to eat at this time in their lives. Do not force them to eat, but attempt to increase dietary fiber and fluids if possible.
2. Mobility: Activity may increase the ability to more easily pass stool. The commode is usually more comfortable than the bedside commode. Avoid the bedpan if at all possible. If the bedpan is the only option, consider using a fracture pan.
3. Drugs: Ask about the patient's drug regimen. Some calcium channel blockers and the tricyclic antidepressants are noted for their ability to constipate. Opioids usually cause constipation.
4. Laxatives: Begin with a "bowel stimulant" such as casanthranol with docusate (Pericolace) or senna (Senekot) in liberal amounts (e.g., 2–4 tabs t.i.d.). A contact laxative (bisacodyl) or an enema might be

needed to start the regimen if the patient has been constipated at the onset. Remember to lubricate the rectum first with a glycerin suppository or oil enema. An osmotic agent such as sorbitol can be added if needed. Usually, no single agent will work alone—it is therefore important to develop a regimen that is appropriate for the individual.[6]

## Ascites

Ascites in the terminally ill person can be asymptomatic. In this case, resist the urge to do something. Symptoms that require intervention include: squashed stomach syndrome, extremity edema, pain from abdominal wall distension, and respiratory compromise. Assuming the underlying cause (e.g., heart failure, liver disease, or malignancy) has been maximally treated, the approach is symptomatic relief. Begin with a paracentesis using an 18G plastic cannula and remove approximately two liters with a suction devise. If vital signs remain stable, some then follow with the use of a gravity drainage bag over the next twelve hours. Spironolactone 200–800mg/day and furosemide 40–80mg/day are the diuretics of choice.[5,6,14] If the person is also troubled by hepatic failure, watch for encephalopathy and treat accordingly.

## ❖ Neurologic

Of all the problems encountered in hospice care, inability to sleep at night and several other disorders, similar in presentation but very different in etiology, cause the greatest deal of distress. The latter include acute confusion, delirium, and terminal restlessness and anxiety. These changes in behavior are seen as suffering by both the lay and professional caregivers and are therefore approached with great angst.

## Sleeplessness

As with all the persons for whom we care, the relief of the symptom(s) causing the patient's distress must be addressed. The most important symptom resulting in sleeplessness is nocturnal pain. The first step in helping the patient overcome sleeplessness is to note if the individual is taking medications or other substances that interfere with sleep—caffeine, steroids, and alcohol. Changes in behavior patterns that can greatly influence nocturnal sleep must also be monitored. These behavior patterns include the person who sleeps during the day, the person who has night fears and is unable to sleep, and the person who is awakened by necessary medical care that results in nocturnal medication or other interventions (e.g., vital signs that interrupt sleep). Management of sleeplessness will depend on the etiology of the problem. Night pain must be controlled. The development of the sustained release opioids has been a major factor in relieving this symptom. Behavior modification is critical. Stimuli to keep the patient awake during the day, psychological approaches to night fears, and even keeping a light on or playing the radio or television might be useful. Finally, medications can be considered. Drugs should only be used for short periods of time and only as needed. The short acting benzodiazepines are the medications of choice. The initial choice would be lorazepam. Remember that many of these individuals are receiving opioids. Increase the nighttime dose two to three times (e.g., if the patient is currently taking sustained release morphine 60mg bid give 90 or 120mg at bedtime in place of the second dose). Nonpharmacologic interventions include massage, a calming presence provided by someone sitting quietly at the bedside, progressive muscle relaxation, visual imagery, or soothing music provided by a bedside cassette tape player.

## *Behavioral Changes*

The change from a mild, quiet person to one who is having hallucinations, gross disorientation, or even more distressing aggressive behavior can lead to total inability of the home caregiver to deal with the patient. The professional can approach this complex situation by recognizing that there is indeed a change in behavior by believing the caregiver that "Dad never acted like this before." Questions to ask in the evaluation of the situation include:

1. Is the patient experiencing any unmet needs (e.g., unrelieved pain, distended bladder, fecal impaction)?
2. Are there any biochemical abnormalities that need to be addressed (e.g., hypercalcemia, azotemia)?
3. Are there any unresolved physical problems (e.g., restraints, uncomfortable bedding)?
4. Are there any unresolved psychological issues (e.g., fear of death, a child or other close family member with whom closure has not been achieved)?
5. Is the patient dealing with any drug induced issues (e.g., antidepressants, stimulants, and withdrawal from alcohol or tobacco)?

Opioids can cause twitching (myoclonic jerking movements) particularly during sleep that may be associated with sleeplessness. Diazepam or lorazepam have been suggested to relieve this twitching as well as muscle spasms and agitated delirium.[22] Therapy is directed toward relieving the etiology of the symptom and the use of specific therapy, if so desired. In this situation, the health care worker may face an ethical dilemma when deciding about treating hypercalcemia and other symptoms in a terminally ill person. When specific therapy is not possible, sedation may be indicated in order to relieve the symptom, not only to alleviate patient distress, but also to relieve family distress.[23] Lorazepam 0.5–1.0mg p.o./s.l. q4–6hrs can be initiated. However, one also needs to consider the use of midazolam 5–240mg/day as a continuous subcutaneous infusion for extremely anxious or restless individuals.[6,12,22–24]

## ❖ Skin

### Pruritus

Pruritus is a common problem among the terminally ill. It is seen in patients diagnosed with leukemia and lymphoma, especially non-Hodgkin's lymphoma. Renal failure is another cause of pruritus. Those patients with hepatic disorders associated with cholestasis may also experience pruritus as a result of blocked bile acids. Some medications, such as morphine sulfate, release histamine which causes pruritus. Pruritus may also be caused by scabies or insect bites. Treatment is based on etiology. The source of the itching should be removed if possible, as in cases of contact dermatitis or drug allergies. Cholestramine resin is helpful in relieving pruritus secondary to partial biliary stasis. However, this medication may make constipation worse. It is relatively expensive and not palatable. Oral antihistamines may be very useful. However, their sedative and drying components must also be considered. General therapeutic measures include cool cloths and emollients applied to damp skin. Care should be taken to avoid soap and lotions that contain perfume and alcohol, since these dry the skin. Lotions and emollients should be applied to damp skin directly after a shower or bath. Hot baths and vasodilators should also be avoided. Simple measures such as clipping the fingernails and applying cotton gloves or socks over the hands may be very helpful in protecting the skin from further injury.[14,25]

### Pressure Ulcers

The terms *decubitus ulcer, pressure sore,* and *pressure ulcer* are often used synonymously. Pressure ulcer is the preferred term because of its accuracy in describing the pathogenesis. The patient's level of mobility or spontaneous movement is the best indicator of risk.[26] A breakdown in skin integrity is common among the terminally ill as mobility decreases and more time is spent in chairs and bed. Treatment is based on the stage of the pressure ulcer. Prevention strategies should be started early. These include maintaining mobility to the fullest extent possible. Bedbound patients should be turned every two hours. Care should be taken to relieve pressure over bony prominence using alternating air mattresses or gel pads. Foam rings should not be used because they increase pressure in one area. Pillows, heel pads, foot cradles, and wedges may be used to reduce pressure on specific areas. Skin should be kept clean of urine and feces using a product which does not dry the skin. Staging guidelines have been developed by the

National Pressure Ulcer Advisory Panel. In Stage I, the skin remains intact, but reddened and nonblanchable. The goal of treatment is to prevent shearing of the skin. In Stage II, the patient experiences a break in skin integrity including partial thickness skin loss involving epidermis and/or dermis. A polyurethane film is recommended for both of these stages. Stage III is defined as full thickness loss of skin including the subcutaneous layer, but not the underlying fascia. The goal in this stage is to protect the wound, promote healing, and prevent infection. A hydrocolloid dressing is recommended if there is little or no exudate. A calcium alginate dressing is recommended for wounds with high levels of exudate. In both cases, the wound should be cleansed with normal saline prior to applying a new dressing. Stage IV pressure ulcers include full thickness skin loss with exposure or destruction of muscle, bone, or other supporting structures. They can include eschar formation and/or infection. The goal of treatment in the terminally ill patient is to prevent or treat infection and keep the pressure ulcer from becoming worse.[27-30]

## Fungating and Ulcerating Malignant Lesions

Management of these lesions includes a thorough assessment beginning with how long the lesion has been present and the effectiveness of previous treatments. As in any other wound, it is also necessary to document the wound's diameter, depth, color, and odor. It is helpful, but not absolutely necessary, to obtain a wound culture. The patient should be queried about physical pain and psychosocial implications surrounding the wound. It is also important to evaluate the patient's support system—who will be responsible for wound care?[31] McMullen found metronidazole to be very effective in controlling odor related to anaerobic bacteria found in fungating malignant lesions and fistulas.[32] The lesions were treated with a topical waterbase gel containing 0.75 percent metronidazole. Fistulas in HIV positive patients were flushed with 1 percent solution containing metronidazole. These treatments resulted in a marked reduction in odor within twenty-four hours. The odor was eliminated within seven days. Pain, edema, and number of dressing changes were dramatically reduced. Newman and colleagues were also successful in treating fungating tumors, pressure sores, and ischemic diabetic lesions and leg ulcers with 0.8 percent metronidazole topical gel.[33] Metronidazole 500mg bid-qid may be administered orally, rectally, vaginally, or intravenously.[11,34] Nonpharmacologic interventions include activated charcoal dressings, yogurt, room deodorizers, and normal saline irrigations.

## ❖ Urinary Tract

Our experience suggests that the three most often encountered urinary problems are failure to initiate flow, painful urination, and bladder spasms. Many of the patients with urinary problems are older men who may have occult prostatic hypertrophy. This can be sufficient to cause failure to empty the bladder. The professional caregiver should also remember to observe for multifactorial etiologies (e.g., debilitation, medications, or physical restraints). Causes of failure to produce urine are beyond the scope of this book. However, the approach to this problem begins by a careful history, since only the patient or caregiver can give this type of information. If the patient has failed to void for twelve hours, there has been only minimal output, or there is the symptom of suprapubic pain or finding a mass in the area, the urinary bladder should be drained using a catheter. If more than 150ml of urine are present, an indwelling catheter is left in place. Depending on the clinical situation this might be all the intervention needed. If the patient is not terminally ill, consider evaluating for reversible conditions. Remember that a full bladder can lead to restlessness.

### Dysuria

Pain on urination is a complaint that is distressing to the patient and should be promptly addressed. The cause of the irritation is most often infection or irritation particularly following instrumentation with a catheter. A topical analgesic such as phenazopyridine (pyridium) 100–200mg t.i.d. should be initiated while awaiting bacterial confirmation.[6,14] Remind the patient that this agent can cause red/orange urine.

### Bladder Spasms

These crampy suprapubic pains are due to the spasmodic contractions of the bladder musculature. The usual cause is irritation due to an indwelling catheter, an obstructed catheter, infection, or fibrosis secondary to therapy (e.g., radiation or cyclophosphamide). The drugs of choice are oxybutynin 5mg t.i.d.; hyoscyamine (Levsin Drops 0.125mg/1ml q4–6hrs sl), or belladonna/opium suppositories q2–4hrs.

### ❖ Lymphedema

The onset of lymphedema is associated with distress because it alters body image and interferes with function of the affected body part. Lymphedema of the upper extremity is usually unilateral being on the same side as the disease process. In the lower extremity it can be either unilateral or bilateral. Causes of unilateral lymphedema include obstruction to flow by cancer or fibrosis secondary to treatment. Etiologies of bilateral edema include problems such as interference in hepatic flow or pelvic lymph node involvement secondary to a malignant process in the region. Under certain circumstances the onset of lymphedema heralds the return of disease (e.g., axillary nodal involvement in breast cancer). The diagnostician is always faced with the dilemma of how and when to evaluate lymphedema. Treatment should be started as early as possible to achieve the best results. Approach the individual with lymphedema with the hope of relieving the problem quickly. Five elements are necessary to optimize care:

1. Active patient involvement. Although this is true for most illnesses, with lymphedema, the patient is also involved in carrying out therapy. The more patients understand about the goals of therapy the more likely they will be an active participant.

2. Skin care. Lymphedema can cause fibrosis in the subcutaneous tissues through an inflammatory response to the edema fluid or secondary to stasis and skin can stretch, leading to breaks in the epidermis causing infection. Optimal skin care requires careful hygiene (e.g., bathing, protective garments when performing activities such as gardening) and attention to lubrication to prevent drying and cracking. Any lubricating lotion applied daily and particularly at night is satisfactory. It is best to avoid perfumed or alcohol-containing products because they dry the skin.

3. Activity of the limb(s). Active or passive range of motion exercises passive or active range of should be tailored for the involved joints because it is important in order to maintain mobility. Immobilizing the extremity leads to further fluid buildup and eventual greater loss of function.

4. Attempt to mobilize the edema using massage therapy and the principles outlined in Badger and Twycross.[35] The essential element of this form of massage is to gently stroke the skin starting in the trunk on the affected side with a motion that barely moves the underlying skin. A more firm stroke will damage the underlying lymphatics and increase the problem. The last area to be drained is the extremity itself, beginning in the proximal regions and proceeding to the distal areas. Pneumatic compression has a role if the lymphedema is severe or has persisted for a period of time. A variety of apparatuses are available and the reader should become familiar with those available in their locale. Venous thrombosis and infection are contraindications to this form of therapy. Congestive heart failure is also a contraindication because of the potential for fluid overload as the edema is shifted from the extremity into the systemic circulation. The possibility of reduced plasma volume, hypotension and altered electrolyte status must also be considered. External support is obtained using elastic hosiery or the equivalent. They must be properly fitted and are best employed as adjuvant to more standard forms of therapy.

## ❖ Summary

It is impossible for people who are dying and plagued by a multitude of symptoms, to be able to do the work necessary to live life until death. With good symptom control the individual is better able to manage the psychosocial issues they face during their illness—especially the good-byes so necessary to achieve closure to both the patient and loved ones.

## ❖ References

1. Grond, S., Zech, D., Diefenbach, C., and Bischoff, A. "Prevalence and Pattern of Symptoms in Patients with Cancer Pain: A Prospective Evaluation of 1635 Cancer Patients Referred to a Pain Clinic." *Journal of Pain and Symptom Management, 9*(6):372–382, 1994.

2. Ahmedzai, S. "Palliation of Respiratory Symptoms." In *Oxford Textbook of Palliative Medicine,* D. Doyle, G. W. C. Hanks, and N. MacDonald, eds. Oxford: Oxford University Press, 1993.

3. Bruera, E., Macmillan, K., Pither, J., and MacDonald, R. N. "Effects of Morphine on the Dyspnea of Terminal Cancer Patients." *Journal of Pain and Symptom Management, 5*:341–344, 1990.

4. Bruera, E., MacEachern, T., Ripamonti, C., and Hanson, J. "Subcutaneous Morphine for Dyspnea in Cancer Patients." *Annals of Internal Medicine, 119*:906–907, 1993.

5. Kaye, P. *Notes on Symptom Control in Hospice and Palliative Care.* Essex: Hospice Education Institute, 1989.

6. Twycross, R. G., and Lack, S. A., eds. *Therapeutics in Terminal Cancer,* 2nd ed. London: Churchill Livingstone, 1990.

7. Storey, P. *Primer of Palliative Care.* Gainesville: Academy of Hospice Physicians, 1994.

8. Farncombe, M., and Chater, S. "Case Studies Outlining Use of Nebulized Morphine for Patients with End-stage Chronic Lung and Cardiac Disease." *Journal of Pain and Symptom Management, 8*:221–225, 1993.

9. Walsh, D. "Dyspnea in Advanced Cancer." *Lancet, 342*:450–451, 1993.

10. McIver, B., Walsh, D., and Nelson, K. "The Use of Chloropromaxine for Symptom Control in Dying Cancer Patients." *Journal of Pain and Symptom Management, 9*:341–345, 1994.

11. Johanson, G. *Physician's Handbook of Symptom Relief in Terminal Care,* 4th ed. Santa Rosa, CA: Sonoma County Academic Foundation for Excellence in Medicine, 1993.

12. Zerwekh, J. V. "Comforting the Dying Dyspneic Patient." *Nursing, 87*:66–69, 1987.

13. Gift, A., Moore, T., and Soeken, K. "Relaxation to Reduce Dyspnea and Anxiety in COPD Patients." *Nursing Research, 4*:242–246, 1992.

14. Woodruff, R. *Palliative Medicine.* Melbourne: Asperula Pty. Ltd., 1993.

15. Alexander, H. R., and Norton, J. A. "Pathophysiology of Cancer Cachexia." In D. Doyle, G. W. C. Hanks, and N. MacDonald, eds. Oxford: Oxford University Press, 1993.

16. Regnard, C., and Fitton, S. "Mouth Care: A Flow Diagram." *Palliative Medicine, 3*:67–69, 1989.

17. Loprinzi, C. L., et al. "Randomized Placebo-Controlled Evaluation of Hydrazine Sulfate in Patients with Advanced Colorectal Cancer." *Journal of Clinical Oncology,* 12:1121–1125, 1994.
18. Chlebowski, R. T., et al. "Hydrazine Sulfate Influence on Nutritional Status and Survival in Non-small Cell Lung Cancer." *Journal of Clinical Oncology,* 8:9–15, 1990.
19. Loprinzi, C. L., et al. "Placebo Controlled Trial of Hydrazine Sulfate in Patients with Newly Diagnosed Non-small-cell Lung Cancer." *Journal of Clinical Oncology,* 12:1125–1129, 1994.
20. Ripamonti, C. "Management of Bowel Obstruction in Advanced Cancer Patients." *Journal of Pain and Symptom Management,* 9(3):193–200, 1994.
21. Mercadante, S., and Maddaloni, S. "Octreotide in the Management of Inoperable Gastrointestinal Obstruction in Terminal Cancer Patients." *Journal of Pain and Symptom Management,* 7(8):496–498, 1992.
22. McNamara, P., Minton, M., and Twycross, R. G. "Use of Midazolam in Palliative Care." *Palliative Medicine,* 5:244–249, 1991.
23. Back, I. N. "Terminal Restlessness in Patients with Advanced Malignant Disease." *Palliative Medicine,* 6:293–298, 1992.
24. Bottomley, D. M., and Hanks, G. W. "Subcutaneous Midazolam Infusion in Palliative Care." *Journal of Pain and Symptom Management,* 5:259–261, 1990.
25. Mortimer, P. S. "Skin Problems in Palliative Care: Medical Aspects." In *Oxford Textbook of Palliative Medicine,* D. Doyle, G. W. C. Hanks, and N. MacDonald, eds. Oxford: Oxford University Press, 1993, pp. 384–395.
26. Low, A. W. "Prevention of Pressure Sores in Patients with Cancer." *Oncology Nursing Forum,* 17(2):179–184, 1990.
27. Levine, J. M., and Totolos, E. "Pressure Ulcers: A Strategic Plan to Prevent and Heal Them." *Geriatrics,* 5:32–37, 1995.
28. Colburn, L. "Pressure Ulcer Prevention for Hospice Patients." *American Journal of Hospice Care,* 4:22–26, 1987.
29. Miller, C. M., O'Neill, A., and Mortimer, P. S. "Skin Problems in Palliative Care: Nursing Aspects."In D. Doyle, G. W. C. Hanks, and N. MacDonald, eds. *Oxford Textbook of Palliative Medicine.* Oxford: Oxford University Press, 1993, pp. 395–407.
30. Panel on the Prediction and Prevention of Pressure Ulcers in Adults. *Pressure Ulcers in Adults: Prediction and Prevention.* AHCPR Publication 92–0047. Rockville, MD: U.S. Department of Health and Human Services, 1992.
31. Gould, D. "Wound Management," *Nursing Mirror,* 159:3–4, 1984.
32. McMullen, D. "Topical Metronidazole Part II." *Ostomy/Wound Management,* 38(3):42–46, 1992.
33. Newman, V., Allwood, M., and Oakes, R. A. "The Use of Metronidazole Gel to Control the Smell of Malodorous Lesions." *Palliative Medicine,* 3:303–305, 1989.
34. Jacob, M. J. "What about Odor in Terminal Cancer?" *Palliative Medicine,* 7(4):31–34, 1991.
35. Badger, C., and Twycross, R. *Management of Lymphedema.* Oxford: Sir Michael Sobell House, 1988.

## ❖ For Further Reading

### General

Bruera, E. "Issues of Symptom Control in Patients with Advanced Cancer." *American Journal of Hospice and Palliative Care*, pp. 12–18, March/April, 1993.

Storey, P. "Symptom Control in Advanced Cancer." *Seminars in Oncology*, 21(6):748–753, 1994.

### Respiratory

de Conno, F., et al. "Does Pharmacological Treatment Affect the Sensation of Breathlessness in Terminal Cancer Patients?" *Palliative Medicine*, 5:237–243, 1991.

Gift, A. "Therapies for Dyspnea Relief." *Holistic Nurse Practice*, 2:57–63, 1993.

### Gastrointestinal

Baines, M., Oliver, D. J., and Carter, R. L. "Medical Management of Intestinal Obstruction in Patients with Advanced Malignant Disease." *Lancet*, pp. 990–993, Nov. 2, 1985.

Canty, S. L. "Constipation as a Side Effect of Opioids." *Oncology Nursing Forum*, 21(4):739–745, 1994.

Haas, F. "In the Patient's Best Interest? Dehydration in Dying Patients." *Professional Nursing*, 10(2):82–87, 1994.

Holden, C. M. "Nutrition and Hydration in the Terminally Ill Cancer Patient: The Nurse's Role in Helping Patients and Families Cope." *The Hospice Journal*, 9(2/3):15–35, 1995.

Kehoe, C. "Malignant Ascites: Etiology, Diagnosis and Treatment." *Oncology Nursing Forum*, 18(3):523–530, 1991.

MacDonald, N. "Cachexia—Anorexia—Asthenia." *Journal of Pain and Symptom Management*, 10(2):151–155, 1995.

Mercandante, S. "Diarrhea in Terminally Ill Patients: Pathophysiology and Treatment." *Journal of Pain and Symptom Management*, 10(4):298–309, 1995.

Mueller, B.A., et al. "Mucositis Management Practices for Hospitalized Patients: National Survey Results." *Journal of Pain and Symptom Management*, 10(7):510–520, 1995.

Regnard, C., and Mannix, K. "Management of Ascites in Advanced Cancer—A Flow Diagram." *Palliative Medicine*, pp. 45–47, 1989.

Sharma, S., and Walsh, D. Management of Symptomatic Malignant Ascites and Diuretics: Two Case Reports and a Review of the Literature. *Journal of Pain and Symptom Management*, 10(3):237–242, 1995.

### Urinary Tract

Smith, P., and Bruera, E. "Management of Malignant Ureteral Obstruction in the Palliative Care Setting." *Journal of Pain and Symptom Management*, 10(6):481–486, 1995.

## ❖ Chapter 10

# Common Questions and Concerns

DENICE C. SHEEHAN

This chapter addresses common questions and concerns regarding hospice care. It is important for the health care worker to understand the concept as well as the services provided by a hospice program in order to have meaningful discussions with terminally ill individuals and their families. The actual services provided by a particular hospice program vary from hospice to hospice even in the same community. The health care worker must explain what each hospice might provide and assist the family in choosing from the available hospices. The information presented in this chapter will provide knowledge about common concerns that will be helpful in discussing hospice and palliative care with the terminally ill, their families, and other health care workers.

Those who want to learn more often call a local hospice or the National Hospice Organization (NHO). In 1994, NHO reported 13,797 telephone and written inquiries. Of these, 3,344 calls were made to the NHO Hospice Helpline.[1] Appendix IIIA lists the Hospice Helpline telephone number as well as the names and addresses of various professional organizations that focus on the care of the dying and bereaved.

## ❖ What Can I Expect?

As more people die in hospitals and extended care facilities rather than at home, fewer people witness the final days and hours of life. Many people have questions about what to expect during the final months, weeks, and days of life. These questions are usually followed by concerns about pain and suffering. Caregivers look to the health care worker for guidance about how they can care for the person who is dying. Although there are predictable clinical signs of impending death, people tend to go through the process of dying as diversely as they progress through life. Death is simply the final stage of life. The apprehension and anxiety experienced by individuals and their families can often be allayed by providing answers to common questions. It is important to listen to the questions and provide appropriate information, being careful to neither evade the question nor overload the person by providing too much information. The individual's culture should also be considered. The health care worker gains a better understanding of the individual's culture and level of participation in that culture by discussing topics such as religious and spiritual beliefs, dietary practices, and cultural and religious rituals. Presumptions based exclusively on generalizations about cultural affiliations negate the importance of the individual's culture-specific needs.[2]

## ❖ Where Will My Loved One Die?

Several myths and misperceptions are associated with hospice care. The first is the concept of hospice as a place where terminally ill individuals go to die. Although the number of hospice facilities is growing as described in Chapter 6, most hospice care is provided in the home.

Second, hospice care is sometimes perceived as hastening death. The fact is, it neither hastens nor delays death. Instead, hospice care provides comfort to the individual and family. This care encompasses the physical, emotional, spiritual, and psychosocial realms in a holistic framework. This final stage of life is not a time to impose change or judgement, but rather a time to support and comfort those who are suffering. Since discomfort and suffering are subjective, the only way to know this about another is to ask and then be willing to listen to the responses.

Enrollment in a hospice program does not necessarily mean the individual must die at home. A 1992 survey conducted by the National Hospice Organizations revealed that 77 percent of the patients died at home, 14 percent died in acute inpatient facilities, and 9 percent in another institution.[3] A recent study of 77 terminally ill patients and their caregivers suggests a correlation between attitudes and place of death. Those who were more realistic and aware that they were dying were more likely to die at home. A home death was also more likely when the family was aware and accepted the prognosis.[4] It is common for the individual and family to vacillate in their preference for a home or hospital death. The interdisciplinary team must realize that the wishes of the individual and family may change over time.

## ❖ Who Will Visit and How Often?

The hospice philosophy defines the patient and family as the unit of care. This differs from other health care models which usually restrict the definition to the patient. Services are provided according to the specific needs of the patient and family members. Decisions regarding the selection of team members and frequency of visits are made by the interdisciplinary team and are outlined in the patient's interdisciplinary plan of care. The Medicare hospice regulations do not require that the patient be homebound. Hospice workers encourage patients to maintain and enhance their quality of life. Therefore, patients may leave their home to visit family, friends, neighbors, shopping malls, or any other outing that interests them. It is sometimes challenging to arrange visits with children who are patients because they often continue to attend school and participate in other activities away from the home. The Medicare hospice regulations do not specify the frequency of home visits. However, they do require the nurse to visit at least every two weeks when home health aide services are being provided. The purpose of these visits is to assess the services of the home health aide.[5]

The hospice nurse is usually the first member of the interdisciplinary team to visit the patient. A visit may be made in the hospital prior to discharge, outpatient clinic, physician's office, or the patient's home on the day the patient leaves the hospital. In some cases this visit is made jointly by the nurse and social worker when there are pressing psychosocial or placement issues. The initial visit is a time to discuss the expectations of the family as well as how those expectations may or may not be able to be met by the hospice team. It is important to listen to the patient's story, sometimes called the history. However, the story is more complex in the hospice setting. Critical information the nurse should obtain includes the patient's perception of the events leading to this day, his or her understanding of the disease process and its impact on quality of life, and past and current treatments with an emphasis on what was and was not helpful. Other questions explore the presence of psychosocial support systems and who will be the primary caregivers. The perceptions of the family are also important. Care should be taken to ensure that people are heard and their concerns are validated. During this visit, the nurse completes a physical assessment and reviews current medications, emphasizing prescription and nonprescription medications as well as vitamins and home remedies. Psychosocial, spiritual, religious, and financial issues are also reviewed. Specific assessment tools may be used to obtain objective data regarding pain, cognitive function, and depression. Examples of these tools are included in Appendix I. Knowledge and skills regarding personal care must be assessed. For example, do the patient and caregiver have the knowledge and manual dexterity to change a colostomy bag or operate an infusion pump for pain control? This baseline information provides the framework for the interdisciplinary plan of care.

Routinely the nurse visits weekly. The frequency of visits may fluctuate depending on the needs of the patient and family. Medicare certified hospices are mandated to provide nursing, pharmacy, and physician services twenty-four hours per day, seven days per week. This is usually accomplished via an on-call telephone system. Most hospice programs employ nurses to triage the telephone calls and make home visits during "off hours." In other programs, the triage nurse assigns the most appropriate team member to make the visit. Many caregivers call at 2 A.M. with a specific physical problem. As the nurse listens, he or she may hear between the lines the need for support and encouragement. Often just knowing someone will answer a call is enough to provide support. In other cases, a home visit is clearly necessary.

Physicians also visit the patient and family at home. The attending physician or hospice medical director may visit at the request of the patient, family, or other member of the interdisciplinary team to evaluate specific concerns or symptoms or attend a family conference.

The social worker visits the patient and family initially. Upon the completion of this assessment, needs of the patient and family are explored and the interdisciplinary plan of care is initiated. This plan may include routine home visits, routine telephone calls, or a combination as needed rather than routinely. Social workers are especially involved in cases where the individual no longer lives at home, or has inadequate finances to pay for expenses. The social worker may also be involved in psychosocial counseling.

The home health aide is requested to visit routinely one to five times per week. These visits are for specific physical care such as bathing, meal preparation, and decubitus care.

The chaplain and/or spiritual care coordinator is available to all patients, but usually does not visit routinely. This is true for the remaining members of the team. The bereavement coordinator may be requested to visit family members who are at high risk for complicated grief or those who are experiencing anticipatory grief. Volunteers are requested for a variety of reasons. In general, a volunteer may do anything that a friend or neighbor may do such as provide respite for the family, take the children to the playground, sit quietly, or engage in stimulating conversation.

## ❖ What Are Family Conferences?

Family conferences are a common vehicle to convey information and develop a plan. They are usually facilitated by the nurse or social worker to enhance communication among family members. Other members of the team may also be invited if they are directly involved in the issues being discussed. Family conferences are convened for many reasons. Some examples are listed in Table 10–1. Family conferences are often held when a family member arrives from another town. The conference provides this person with the opportunity to ask questions and to participate in the discussion about the patient's care. Patients often request the presence of several family

TABLE 10–1    Reasons for Family Conferences

To discuss progression of disease

To discuss the home environment

To discuss expectations of hospice and of family

To discuss feelings (e.g., incompetence, anxiety, worry, feeling overwhelmed)

To discuss moving the patient to a different residence

To facilitate communication between patient and family members

To discuss self care for the caregiver (e.g., taking breaks, meeting own needs)

members to discuss the progression of disease and what to expect in the near future. In a situation where the patient, family, or hospice team perceives the patient to be in an unsafe environment, a family conference may be convened to discuss these concerns and possibly discuss other living arrangements. A family conference may also be held to discuss the unmet expectations of the patient and family. Family members often express feelings of incompetence. They may feel overwhelmed in caring for the patient. The combination of teaching skills and offering support through a conference can be very helpful. Respite options may also be discussed at this time.

## ❖ What Medications, Supplies, and Equipment Will Be Provided?

All hospice services, durable medical equipment, supplies, and medications needed for the palliation and management of the terminal illness and related conditions are fully covered under the Medicare hospice benefit and many other private insurance companies. The interdisciplinary plan of care provides the framework within which to determine the appropriateness of specific services, equipment, supplies, medications, tests, and treatments. Chapter 2 provides more details about reimbursement for hospice care.

The initial assessment often reveals a myriad of medications from several different medical specialists in addition to nonprescription medicines and home remedies. Often neither the patient nor the family are knowledgeable about the rationale, dose, or side effects of the medications. The nurse, physician, and pharmacist work together to provide optimum medications. The guidelines for choosing the most appropriate medication include multiple benefits, minimal side effects, ease of administration and cost. Some individuals are unable to afford their medications, equipment and supplies. The hospice nurse is knowledgeable about community resources. For example, many pharmaceutical companies offer indigent care programs and the American Cancer Society offers medical equipment and supplies to those with cancer.

## ❖ What to Do during an Emergency?

An emergency may be defined as a situation requiring immediate attention. The perceptions of the people experiencing the emergency and their coping strategies will determine their response. Often talking with a hospice worker will help put the person's concerns into perspective in order to decide upon appropriate actions. Caregivers usually call hospice when sudden changes occur. These include restlessness, increased pain, difficulty in breathing, and agitation. Explaining the cause of these changes is of tremendous help to the patient and family. Specific instructions may be given by telephone. A home visit may be necessary to determine the cause and appropriate interventions or to provide support.

## ❖ What Happens When Death Approaches?

Health care workers and other caregivers are often at a loss for specific ways to provide comfort for the terminally ill individual. Sitting next to the patient who is in a bed or chair is very important. This sends a quiet message to the individual that he or she is cherished. The simple act of being is often more important than doing. Encouraging the individual to participate in life review is helpful. Everyone has a story to tell which is individually unique and can only be told by that person. Reminiscent therapy as life review is complemented by sharing pictures and relating them to specific memories, people, and places. An avid reader appreciates a story being read aloud or an audiotape player for recorded books. These are available from community libraries and agencies that work with the blind.

Terminally ill individuals often experience the appearance of family members and friends who have already died. Often religious figures are seen in the room. Patients may talk to these people or hold out their arms to them. These experiences are usually very peaceful and calming to the individual. However they can upset the family. It is helpful to the individual to validate these experiences and to reassure the family that these are common experiences. Some people talk about wanting to go home when they are at home. It is helpful to explore the meaning behind the words. The words "going home" might mean "to die." The authors of *Final Gifts* explore the use of metaphors and various communication techniques used by those who are dying. This is done through the use of scenarios from their clinical practice as hospice nurses.[6]

As the person enters the final phase of living, there is usually a decrease in appetite, thirst, and urinary output. This is a natural adaptive process. The body is no longer able to assimilate food and fluids. It is normal for urinary output to become more concentrated and decrease in quantity. This is usually the result of decreased intake and renal function as multisystem failure progresses. Feeding and hydration issues become very important during the final phase of life. This is especially true for those who link nurturing and love with food and drink. It is important to explore other ways to nurture and share love. Forcing food and drink may cause discomfort for the individual. Aspiration may occur if the person has difficulty swallowing. Thirst and dry mouth are common sources of discomfort. Ice chips, popsicles, small sips of fluid and water soluble lubricants keep the mouth and lips moist. Many caregivers will be worried when peripheral edema occurs. It is important to carefully explain that this is a common finding when multi-organ systems fail.

The individual may spend more time sleeping or prefer to be alone much of the time. It is common for socialization to decrease during this time of life when energy is limited and one is no longer expected to socialize. Energy is conserved by pulling inward. This energy is needed to maintain basic circulatory and respiratory functions.

It is common for breathing patterns to change. The person may experience rapid shallow breathing or periods of apnea followed by several deep breaths. Noisy tachypnea may be present in the dying person. Noisy rattling respirations are heard as the secretions move up and down at the back of the throat with inspiration and expiration.

Often an individual seems to be on the verge of death, but unable to die. This person may be worried about those he or she leaves behind. The family may need guidance to say goodbye and give permission to the person to die. This closure can be very helpful to both the dying person and those saying goodbye.

## ❖ What to Do at the Time of Death?

It is important for the physician or nurse to discuss the signs of imminent death with the caregiver. These are listed in Table 10–2. Some people will experience all signs and symptoms while others will experience none of them. Caregivers are instructed and encouraged to call hospice at the time of death. A home visit is offered at this time. If accepted, the nurse makes this visit and examines the patient. Depending on state law, the nurse or physician may determine that the patient is dead. If a nurse or physician is not called, the coroner may need to be notified at the time of death. If the family calls the local emergency medical services (EMS), they may be obligated to contact the police if the person is dead and a physician or nurse has not made a visit. If the patient is alive when they arrive, the individual may be transported to the nearest hospital, even though the person is actively dying. This transport may be appropriate if the patient or family prefers that the patient die in the hospital. It is important to be sensitive to religious and cultural beliefs of the family. Instructions regarding autopsy and organ donation should also be followed. Specific protocols need to be followed in cases of organ donation. The nurse may prepare the patient's body for transport to the funeral home by removing various medical supplies such as a foley catheter or nasal cannula and cleaning the body. Family members may be invited to assist in this preparation. Other members of the interdisciplinary team may be present at the time of death. It is appropriate for any team member to support the family by listening, answering questions, and offering assistance with specific tasks such as arranging for the transport of the patient's body to the funeral home. This is also an excellent opportunity for

TABLE 10–2   Signs of Imminent Death

Cold, mottled skin

Periods of apnea

Decreased or no urine output

Decreased level of consciousness

Bowel and/or bladder incontinence

Increased somnolence

the hospice worker to assess those present for signs of high risk for complicated grief. Bereavement counseling is offered for one year after the death. The type and frequency of support is dependent on the level of need.

## ❖ Summary

Hospice programs provide a wide range of services based on the needs of the patient and family. It is important to determine the expectations of the patient and family prior to initiating hospice services. It is also necessary to continue to explore these expectations so that specific needs may be met by the appropriate resources. Questions and concerns should be identified and discussed as they arise. It is comforting for patients and families to know what to expect and how hospice workers can support them during this journey.

## ❖ References

1. National Hospice Organization. *Newsline,* Feb. 15, 1995.
2. Pickett, M. "Cultural Awareness in the Context of Terminal Illness." *Cancer Nursing, 16*(2):102–106, 1993
3. National Hospice Organization. "National Hospice Profile." *Newsline,* Oct. 1993.
4. Hinton, J. "Which Patients with Terminal Cancer are Admitted from Home Care?" *Palliative Medicine, 8*(3):197–210, 1994
5. U.S. Department of Health and Human Services. *Medicare: Hospice Manual, Rev.* U.S. Department of Health and Human Services. Washington, DC: U.S. Department of Commerce National Technical Information Service, 1992.
6. Callanan, M., and Kelley, P. *Final Gifts: Understanding the Special Awareness, Needs and Communications of the Dying.* New York: Poseidon Press, 1992.

## ❖ For Further Reading

Holden, C.M. "Easing the Burden of Decision Making in Futile Situations." *Health Care Ethics Committee Forum, 7*(5):322–330, 1995.
Lindley-Davis, B. "Process of Dying." *Cancer Nursing, 14*(6):328–333, 1991.

# ❖ Chapter 11

# Death Education: Teaching Staff, Patients, and Families about the Dying Process

Lauren R. Zeefe

This chapter will explore death education within a hospice program. The objective of this chapter is to enhance the understanding of the dying process in order to understand the issues raised when confronting death. Some of these issues are listed in Table 11–1.

Death education deals with the process of death and dying, including bereavement. Those who teach about death address topics such as attitudes concerning death in culture and society (e.g., fear and denial of death); the grieving process; customs and rituals, including the burial process; evaluating interventions which effect the process when they interfere with the functioning of those still living. Death education has been defined as a term which applies to a wide variety of planned educational experiences that improve knowledge and understanding of the meaning of death, the process of dying, and grief and bereavement.[1] Death education involves formal as well as informal teaching. Although there are frequent reminders that death remains a taboo and fearful topic for many people, there is evidence that our society is in a period of transition. Death education encompasses formal instruction dealing with dying, death and grief, and informal exploration of these topics. "Teachable moments" arising out of death-related events occurring in daily life provide excellent opportunities for death education in an informal context.[2] Ongoing education enhances bereavement programs and advances professional development in hospice care. Death education,

TABLE 11–1    Points to Ponder When Discussing Dying

Understanding the emotional changes that occur during the dying process

Becoming aware of the physical changes that occur during the dying process

Recognizing the reactions to the death of an individual or loved one

Dealing with the special needs of the dying

Identifying abnormal reactions to the dying process either for staff or family

Understanding one's own reaction to the dying process

Offering the opportunity for growth during the dying process designed specifically through educational programs and presentations, can provide ongoing opportunities for bereavement care. Death education can enhance hospice services in the community by providing opportunities to:

Identify, develop, and enhance bereavement practices in support of the terminally ill and their families.

Develop and strengthen skills of hospice and other health care professionals regarding bereavement and loss.

## ❖ Death Education for Staff

Fundamental skills are required for the professional dealing with the dying and the bereaved. Attitudes, skills, and knowledge are critical for the staff as they face the grief process and the tasks that families in mourning must confront. Death education assists the hospice team members to recognize and normalize dying, as well as the grief process. Humanistic empathetic attitudes, communicative and listening skills are part of the development that occurs through death education. The goals of death education often reflect the needs of the staff and the family.[1] Societal anxiety regarding death often anesthetizes the experience of loss and prohibits discussion and movement between staff, patient, and family. It is important, then, for the staff to feel comfortable with the knowledge that death is a natural part of the life cycle. For the hospice staff addressing issues of death, death education is beneficial in understanding the physical and psychosocial challenges of the dying process objectively and subjectively.[2] Death education is a process that occurs over time. Thus, it is necessary to train hospice professionals in death education on a continuing basis, as part of their daily activities. New hospice employees generally attend a well defined and rigorous orientation. Basic components of death education which should be included in the orientation program are listed in Table 11–2.

Bereavement services are mandated by the Medicare hospice regulations.[3] These services are provided for up to one year after the death of the patient. A

Table 11–2    Hospice Orientation Program Death Education Components

---

1.  Introduction and overview of the field
2.  Basic theories of grief and bereavement
    a.  Erich Lindemann—Symptomatology of Acute Grief
    b.  Colin Murray Parkes—Defined Stages of Grief
3.  Types of grief
4.  Approaches to helping the bereaved
5.  Discussion of children and bereavement
6.  Visit to a mortuary
7.  General review, discussion and role playing

---

Source: Corr, C. A., and Corr, D. M. *Hospice Care Principles and Practice*. Springer Publishing Co., 1983.

bereavement coordinator, usually a social worker, nurse, or psychologist, must establish clear goals and objectives for the program to be successful. A hospice bereavement program often uses trained volunteers to help with the continuity of aftercare services. Again, like staff, volunteers are required to attend orientation and training in bereavement. A solid conceptual framework of knowledge about bereavement, grief, and mourning is currently provided through education. This training prepares professionals to assist the bereaved in a preventative and health-promoting manner, and to support them during the process of grieving for their losses. Often they are able to make and promote appropriate referrals or suggest other interventions. The goal of this work is to achieve the most constructive resolution possible.[4]

## ❖ Death Education for Patients and Families by Staff

Hospice team members teach individuals and families about the death and dying process with support and compassion. Team members also learn from their clients and their families. Hospice workers often have the opportunity to assist families prior to the patient's death. They may support and educate the members of the family, and observe family functioning in order to plan for effective follow-up.[5] The dying person faces several tasks.[6] The individual must arrange a variety of affairs, which requires the acknowledgement of his or her impending death. Hospice staff encourage individuals and families to continue to behave with as much autonomy and control as possible. When this task seems too difficult for the individual and their family, the hospice team members can explore issues that might prevent or retard the task from being carried out. Helping the individual and family to understand the disease process and maintain symptom and pain control can help alleviate fear. Thus, they might be able to maintain control so that unfinished business can be attended. The dying person must undertake the task of coping with loss, both of loved ones and the self. This task questions the effect that the death will have on the loved ones, as well as one's own loss. Here is a critical moment when the hospice staff can intervene by using skills that will allow both the individual and family to open lines of communication and strengthen family bonds. It is common for them to ignore the dying process in order to protect one another. Staff can be especially helpful when they understand that the grieving process can begin prior to the death. The anticipated loss known as anticipatory grief is a form of normal grieving. The dying person must see to future medical care needs, which allows the person to exercise some type of control regarding the plan of care. Hospice staff can help the dying person and caregiver with concrete skills and information. What arrangements are to be made when the patient is no longer capable? The hospice staff can utilize their skills while treading on delicate waters. The hospice team member can explain living wills and advance directives to the patient and the family, allowing wishes to be fulfilled whenever possible. The dying person must cope effectively with the loss of self, as well as death. Hospice personnel can support the patient and the family facing death. Understanding that grief is a process and not an event, the staff can offer information and insight into the process of dying to offer some sense of reason. Reason, in turn, attempts to restore order when the impact of terminal illness has splintered the lives of a family. A collaborative relationship between staff and patient/family can effectively render coping skills that will help with the grieving process.

## ❖ Society and Death Education

Death education can provide a framework for understanding issues in society concerning death and the dying process. Death education can address the following issues facing contemporary society: integrating death and dying into the social structure particularly important in an aging society; developing appropriate support systems, which include the necessary rituals; and understanding the full impact of matters such as physician assisted suicide and euthanasia. All these concerns will continue to challenge our social fabric. There seems to be three general patterns of response for all societies: death-accepting, death-defying, or death-denying.[7] Regardless of the pattern that society embraces, education can help facilitate a greater and more significant understanding of loss. Some basic goals of understanding issues of death and dying in society include:

1. A greater awareness of our own feelings regarding loss, leading to a deeper sense of empathy and compassion.
2. An understanding of the grief process and experience.
3. A normalization of death and dying.
4. Diminished fears of death and dying.
5. Societal attitudes, reform, and acceptance within a diverse population.
6. Educational development to act as a springboard for issues regarding informed consent and advance directives.

Death education in hospice addresses these issues with staff, the dying person, and their family. Applied to the community, it can be an essential component for helping society understand issues of death and dying as well. Programs by hospice personnel that explain the dying process, teach about grieving and complicated mourning, and explain the various ethnic or religious customs will assist society to be better prepared to accept the concepts espoused by death education. In particular, the isolation of the dying person, abolishing fears such as all death is painful, and dispelling myths that often surround a dying person are all areas where the hospice staff can assist the community in learning to cope. The bereaved are especially affected by the lack of death education in the community. Pressure from a poorly informed public can force a grieving individual to reenter "normal activities" before the grieving process has progressed to the point where this is feasible. The consequences of this can produce behavioral changes, somatic complaints, and poor work performance that could have been avoided. Thus, death education by hospice professionals validates the bereaved by educating the public on the normal aspects of grief, including the various idiosyncratic reactions that individuals might exhibit. For example, elderly men who are widowed are at risk for early death following the death of the spouse. Longer life span, which has occurred in this century, poses new problems for society. While modern treatment and technology can offer options, they cannot suspend death. Death education is becoming a part of university curricula. Trained professionals are available to lead workshops and seminars. The National Hospice Organization (NHO) maintains a list of speakers. With a deeper understanding of death and dying issues, we as a society can realize and recognize the normality of death. Death education offers a platform in which society can gain a greater awareness and a deeper understanding of people facing the death of a loved one.

## ❖ Facing Death: Issues for the Individual and Hospice Staff

When do we begin to die? The following possibilities have been suggested:

1. Dying begins the moment we are born.
2. Dying begins when a fatal condition begins.
3. Dying begins when a fatal condition is recognized by a physician.
4. Dying begins when the patient is told that his or her condition is fatal.
5. Dying begins when the patient realizes and accepts the facts.
6. Dying begins when nothing more can be done to reverse the condition and preserve life.[1]

It has become increasingly apparent that health professionals play an important role in helping individuals face death. Although death education can assist in a greater awareness and understanding of death and dying, it cannot predict or control one's reaction to impending death. Facing death means separation, letting go. This extraordinary task is not always gracefully achieved between the dying person and the family. Certain coping techniques such as denial can become unhealthy and interfere with the opportunity for good-byes and new growth during the dying process. However, it is important to recognize that there is not a right or wrong way to accept death or a right or wrong way to die. Every death, like every person, is unique and individual. Rando has suggested that individuals face seven tasks of dying.[6] These are listed in Table 11–3. During this critical time hospice staff can intervene and enhance or open the line of communication between the individual and the family. However, a family system can be open or closed, so it is important to strive for the promotion of communication to the extent that the individual and family permit.[7] It is evident that the dying person and their family encounter stress, fear, pain, suffering, loneliness, isolation, loss of body image, loss of independence, separation, anxiety, financial burden, and possibly loss of hope and/or meaning. Hospice staff can help patients and family understand some of these concerns and

TABLE 11–3   Seven Tasks of Dying

1. Dealing with discomfort, incapacitation, and other symptoms of the illness or injury itself

2. The management of the stresses of special treatment procedures and the institutional setting itself

3. Developing and maintaining adequate relationships with caregivers

4. Preserving a reasonable emotional balance by managing upsetting feelings aroused by the illness, such as anxiety, anger, alienation, inadequacy, or guilt

5. Preserving a satisfactory self-image and maintaining a sense of competence and mastery

6. Preserving relationships with family and friends

7. Preparing for an uncertain future in which significant losses are  threatened

Source: Rando, T. A. Grief, Dying, and Death Clinical Interventions for Caregivers. Research Press Company, 1984.

teach them to modify effective coping skills to meet their needs. Facing death can also cause a spiritual crisis. For some, when cure is no longer an option, spiritual and/or religious beliefs become strong comfort measures. Grief responses and mourning rituals and customs are unique and diverse. The hospice philosophy does not impose any particular religious or spiritual values upon the dying person. It seeks the opportunity to assist the patient to actualize any spiritual values the patient may hold.[1]

Diversity has been defined as the valorization of alternate lifestyles, biculturality, human differences, and uniqueness in individual and group life.[7] Diversity may include but not be limited to African Americans, Pacific Islander/Asian Americans, American natives, children, persons with AIDS, a religious group, and others. Hospice workers are advised to stop, listen, and learn about each other, and about each patient, family, culture, and community in order to improve the care of the dying. When facing the prospects of involvement in death education, it is critical to include a cross-cultural component to clarify values, beliefs, and customs, and heighten the sensitivity and awareness of the staff toward these differences. The hospice staff will encounter barriers when working with diverse populations. Whether it be language, customs, religious beliefs, or approach to various medical treatments, if these barriers are not properly understood and identified, they will impede effective hospice services. Components of understanding the cultural barriers include both formal and informal teaching.[8] An understanding of basic concepts is necessary to understand the essence of culturally relevant care. Culture describes the total body of beliefs, behaviors, sanctions, values, and goals that marks the way of life of any people. Tucker and Harris suggest that certain skills and concepts be learned in order to develop a plan of care that is culturally sensitive when persons are facing death.[9] These are listed in Table 11–4. Developing culturally-sensitive death education programs enhances our understanding of fears, anxiety, expectations, perceptions, assumptions, definitions, prejudices, emotions, and attitudes.

TABLE 11–4  Skills and Concepts Needed to Develop a Culturally Sensitive Plan of Care for Hospice Patients

Cultural identity and spiritual needs

Staff and patient roles

Values clarification

Group characteristics (ethics)

Nutritional assessment of cultural groups

Health problems of at-risk population groups

Differences between providers' and consumers' views of health-related matters

Interventions for clients from different cultures

Use of cultural assessment tools

*Source:* Tuck, I., and Harris, L. "Teaching Students Transcultural Concepts." *Nurse Educator,* 13(3):36–39, 1988.

TABLE 11–5  Clinical Signs in the Dying Patient

Increasing somnolence and progressing to unresponsiveness

Periods of apnea

Mottled and cold skin

Decreasing oral intake and urinary output

Loss of involuntary muscle control

Gurgling

## *Clinical Signs in the Dying Patient*

It is often helpful to anticipate questions from the family about the dying process. Although it is difficult to anticipate what signs are associated with dying, several are prominent. These are listed in Table 11–5. One system of scoring progression of disease used in the oncology setting is the Karnofsky Score.[9] This score, coupled with an evaluation of other factors such as nutritional status, activities of daily living, comorbid conditions particularly in the elderly, and even emotional status will assist the hospice professional to better estimate survival. However, as is clear to all who have tried to predict survival, this effort is often inaccurate.

## ❖ Summary

The challenge and significance of death education in hospice is to develop, enhance and maintain the skills, practices, and relationships of interdisciplinary teams, terminally ill persons, and families facing the impact of death and the associated bereavement. Death education should be an ongoing process that permits individuals continued development and growth in bereavement. The commitment of death education in hospice provides a greater awareness and experience of death and dying issues. Death education also offers opportunity for growth and development for staff, the dying, and their families during the last stages of life. Death education can assure the individual and the family facing death that unequaled care was given, thus reducing stress and guilt and bestowing equanimity.

## ❖ References

1. Kastenbaum, R., and Kastenbaum, B. *Encyclopedia of Death. Myth, History, Philosophy, Science—The Many Aspects of Death and Dying.* New York: Avon Books, 1989.
2. DeSpelder, L. A., and Strickland, A. L. *The Last Dance. Encountering Death and Dying.* Mountain View, CA: Mayfield Publishing Company, 1992.
3. Osterweis, M., Solomon, F., and Green, M. *Bereavement Reactions, Consequences and Care.* Washington, DC: National Academy Press, 1984.
4. U.S. Department of Health and Human Services, *Medicare: Hospice Manual, Rev.* U.S. Department of Health and Human Services. Washington, DC: U.S. Department of Commerce National Technical Information Service, 1992.
5. Kalish, R. A. "The Onset of the Dying Process." *Omega*, 57–69, 1970.
6. Rando, T. A. *Grief, Dying, and Death Clinical Interventions for Caregivers.* Champaign, IL: Research Press Company, 1984.
7. Harper, B. C. *Caring For Our Own With Respect, Dignity and Love The Hospice Way.* A Handbook for Inclusive Care from the National Hospice Organization's Task Force on Access to Hospice Care by Minorities. Arlington, VA: National Hospice Organization, 1994.
8. Tuck, I., and Harris, L. "Teaching Students Transcultural Concepts." *Nurse Educator, 13*(3): 1988.
9. Mor, V., et al. "The Karnofsky Performance Scale: An Examination of Its Reliability and Validity in a Research Setting." *Cancer, 53*:2002–2007, 1984.

## ❖ For Further Reading

Beresford, L. *The Hospice Handbook.* Boston: Little, Brown and Company, 1993.
Corless, I. B., Germino, B. B., and Pittman, M., eds. *Dying, Death, and Bereavement: Theoretical Perspectives and Other Ways of Knowing.* Boston: Jones and Bartlett, 1994.
Kirschling, J. M., and Osmont, K. "Bereavement Network: A Community Based Group." *Omega, 27*(2):119–127, 1993.
Longman, A. J. "Effectiveness of a Hospice Community Bereavement Program." *Omega, 27*(2):165–175, 1993.
Rando, T. A. *Treatment of Complicated Mourning.* Champaign, IL: Research Press, 1993.
Sammarino, D. "Acute Care Patients vs. Terminally Ill Patients." *Thanatology Newsletter, 1*(4): 1992.

# ❖ Chapter 12

# Ethical Issues in Hospice Care

DAVID BARNARD

Health care is essentially a moral enterprise. Every clinical encounter is influenced by the personal and cultural values of both the patient and the provider, the moral traditions of the health professions, and the social and political contexts of the health care system. Many of the ethical issues that arise in the care of the dying, therefore, are similar to issues that arise in many other areas of health care: truthfulness and confidentiality; decision-making authority in the professional-patient relationship; and the appropriate use and allocation of technology and other health care resources. Other issues are more commonly associated with the care of the terminally ill, though not absent from other arenas—decisions to withhold or withdraw life-sustaining treatment; decision making for patients who have lost their own decision-making capacity; requests for assistance in suicide or active euthanasia.

Two other factors assure the need for moral reflection in palliative care. First, most professionals who enter the field do so because they want to help people die well. But what does it mean to "die well?" What is a "good death?" There is no single, universal answer to these questions. Even with respect to elements of a "good death" on which most people could probably agree—freedom from pain, resolution of personal affairs, the supportive presence of loved ones—there is room for considerable personal variation. People differ in how they balance pain relief against alertness; in their willingness to face the reality of their imminent death; in their desire to talk about their feelings to friends, family, or caregivers; and in their willingness to tolerate increasing weakness, dependency, and uncertainty rather than trying to control the timing and manner of their death through an act of suicide or euthanasia. This variability requires health professionals to approach patients and families as individuals, and attempt to provide care that is consistent both with patient and family values and with their own conscience.

Second, the approach of death and loss is profoundly stressful for patients, families, and caregivers. And yet, in this atmosphere of stress, anxiety, fear, and grief, decisions must continually be made about complex matters of pain and symptom control, the use of diagnostic tests, how much to tell whom about what, and so on. Clarity about the moral dimensions of these decisions, and about the factors one ought to take into account, can be of great help to all involved.

A chapter of this size cannot address all of the ethical issues in hospice and palliative care. Rather, it emphasizes issues that are most likely to arise in everyday practice. Discussion of these topics will emphasize ethical and clinical considerations that apply to other issues as well. While there is as yet no comprehensive book-length treatment of ethics in palliative care, the *Journal of Palliative Care* has recently devoted two special thematic issues to this subject in Volume 10, Numbers 2 and 3, 1994.

### ❖ Expectations of Patients, Family, and Team

Hospice and palliative care is appropriate when a patient's disease is no longer amenable to cure, when prolongation of life is no longer the goal, and when maximizing the patient's comfort and quality of life takes precedence over other objectives. Ideally, a patient or family's decision to enter hospice care is the result of an open, deliberate decision-making process in which the goals and expectations of patient, family, and professional team are closely matched. Unfortunately, this is not always the case. Some patients may be referred to hospice without adequate preparation by the referring physician. Sometimes the referring physician will have provided a full explanation of the limitations of curative treatment and the options for palliative care, but patient or family's denial will have prevented the physician's message from getting through. Sometimes expectations are unclear because the patient's clinical status is unclear. The distinction between acute, curative care, and palliative care is not always obvious. The transition from curative to palliative goals is often a gradual process, full of clinical uncertainty and ambivalence on both sides of the professional-patient relationship.

For all of these reasons, it is important to assess and clarify goals and expectations from the very beginning of the relationship between the patient, family, and hospice team. The team needs to know as much as possible about the patient's previous clinical course, and equally important, *what the patient and family have been told*, and *what they appear to understand* about that course. Medical records are often seriously deficient in recording the details and nuances of a patient's understanding of his or her disease. The cursory notation, "Patient and family educated about the situation," can mask a host of ambiguities and distortions. These problems are less likely to occur if the hospice team has been following the patient on a consultative basis for a period of time before taking full clinical responsibility for the patient, but this situation is relatively rare. More often the team will need to familiarize itself with the patient's situation on short notice, and clear communication with the referring physician is essential. The new relationship between the hospice team and the patient and family is most likely to get off on the right foot when ambiguities in the patient's understanding are identified and clarified as soon as possible. Even when the philosophy and goals of hospice and palliative care are generally understood and accepted, divergent expectations can emerge in interactions with the patient or family around a number of specific issues. Two of the most common are the communication of information about the patient's condition—to the family or to the patient him- or herself—and the management of pain, especially with narcotic analgesics.

## Communication of Information

Open and forthright communication about diagnostic and prognostic information has become a widely accepted norm in health care over the past twenty-five years. This contrasts with a more paternalistic past in which communication about "bad news" was routinely avoided in order to protect patients from the distressing impact of such information. There is now a greater understanding that deception and the "conspiracy of silence" are likely to cause more harm to the patient and family than the information itself. As a result, discussions of truthtelling in health care have shifted from the question *whether* to disclose bad news to the questions *how, when, to whom,* and *how often* to disclose it.[1,2]

Nevertheless, even in the hospice and palliative care setting where open acknowledgment of dying, death, and grief is regarded as a cardinal virtue, the team is occasionally faced with conflicts over the issue of truthfulness and information control. They may encounter families who insist that information regarding diagnosis or prognosis be withheld from the patient, or, conversely, patients who demand that their relatives not be told the truth about their condition.[3] The latter situation has become more common recently with patients who are dying of AIDS.

In responding to patients or family members who insist that information be withheld from others who, in the judgment of the team, ought to have that information, it is important to remember the *individuality* of patients and families. Pat answers or doctrinaire moralizing are inappropriate. Each request or demand should be treated sympathetically and with respect, but each should also be assessed thoroughly. *Why* does the family member, for example, believe that the patient should not be given more information about her or his situation? What *specific harms* does the family member foresee as consequences of more open communication? Is there any *evidence from the past* that supports the family member's concerns? Questions such as these, asked in a sympathetic and understanding manner, may elicit valuable information, including greater awareness of cultural factors that should indeed be taken into account in communicating with the patient. More commonly, these questions will give the team the opportunity to allay the family member's own anxieties and open the way to freer communication with the patient.

The team can recount wide experience that patients typically understand more of the truth of their situation than family members suspect; that restricted communication and conspiracies of silence tend to increase the patient's sense of isolation at the very time connectedness and intimacy are most important;

and that the relief that comes from mutual recognition of the patient's situation can lead to very meaningful family interactions, and can contribute to the family's ability to make the most of the time they have left together.[4,5,6] Finally, the team can offer to help with communication by being present at key moments, or by taking the lead in introducing a difficult topic. A similar, individualized approach should be taken with patients who request that information about their condition should be withheld from family members.

Communication of information about illness and prognosis is a *process*. It is not a once and done event. Patients and families move in and out of direct awareness of threatening information. Periods of denial can be protective, allowing threatening information to be absorbed gradually.[7,8,9] Conversations will likely have to be repeated several times. Similarly, a family member or a patient who initially insists that information be withheld may change his or her position as time goes by. This is another reason not to respond confrontationally to the initial request—to preserve a supportive relationship that can facilitate change over time.

## Pain Management

Particularly in the management of patients at home, patient or family attitudes toward the use of narcotic analgesics can be a source of frustration and ethical concern for the hospice team. Patient stoicism, fears of addiction, fear that admitting to pain means admitting that the disease has progressed, or reluctance to tolerate side effects can all lead patients or families to resist analgesic medications, leaving the patient in pain. As in the case of communication of information, a sympathetic assessment of patient and family concerns is the best course to follow at the outset.

The team can address misconceptions about addiction. Medication, dosage, or route of administration can be adjusted to minimize side effects.[10] It is important to ascertain the patient's own preferences regarding the trade-off between drowsiness and pain relief—a common issue in the use of opioids. While the goal is maximum pain control *and* maximum alertness, some balancing is usually necessary, and the patient is the person who—if he or she is able—should strike the balance for him or herself.

More difficult problems arise in cases where patients depend on family members to receive their pain medications, and the family is withholding the medication for reasons of their own. Some patients may be excellent candidates for continuous subcutaneous analgesia, via a portable syringe driver, to obviate the need for family member involvement in the administration of the medication. Yet some family members may refuse to allow the syringe driver to be applied, again out of fear that this would be a sign of advancing disease, or out of frustration at losing control of yet one more aspect of the patient's care.

In these situations, which fortunately are relatively infrequent, the family members' anxieties and concerns need to be addressed sympathetically and directly. Often, simply giving the opportunity to ventilate fears and frustrations leads to a greater spirit of cooperation in the management of the patient's pain. In other cases it may be useful to admit the patient for a period of inpatient care (if appropriate facilities are available). This can serve at least two important purposes. First, it allows the team more direct observation and control of the patient's experience of pain. Second, it provides the family with respite from the heavy demands of caregiving. This may be crucial in allowing the family to face the patient's situation more realistically, and help them participate more constructively in the patient's care, when and if he or she returns home.

There are rare and extreme situations where the hospice team believes a nonautonomous, dependent patient is suffering extreme pain because of family members' inability or unwillingness to cooperate in pain management. In such situations more drastic and forceful interventions may have to be considered. These may include invoking abuse and neglect statutes under state law, institutionalization of the patient, and judicial appointment of a guardian for the purposes of accepting recommended medical treatment. Because such measures are so intrusive and adversarial, however, and introduce the impersonal mechanisms of the court system into the deeply personal and intimate context of a family's encounter with death, they should be considered a last, desperate resort. They may have a limited role, but only when all other measures have failed, and the risks of grave harm to the patient seem otherwise unavoidable.

## General Considerations in Managing Conflicting Expectations among Patients, Families, and Team

Communication and pain management are but two of a variety of issues around which patients, families, and hospice and palliative care teams can experience conflicting expectations. Other important issues that cannot be thoroughly discussed for reasons of space, include expectations regarding how aggressively to diagnose or treat problems that arise in the terminal phase (e.g., dyspnea, dysphagia, anorexia, renal insufficiency, bowel obstruction, or fever). Even when all agree that the patient's comfort is the chief concern, not prolongation of life, there is room for uncertainty about the appropriate response to these problems in particular situations. As in each of the preceding sections, a sympathetic, individualized approach is indicated in response to patient or family inquiries about available interventions. It is important to avoid simply falling back on sweeping statements such as, "We don't do that in palliative care," or "That would be inconsistent with the goals of hospice," without a careful assessment of the individual circumstances and the motivations behind the inquiry.[11,12]

Individualized care and sympathetic responses to patients and families are the most important general considerations in managing and minimizing conflicting expectations. There are several other points to keep in mind as well.

First, in evaluating and responding to family expectations, it is essential to remember the family's crucial roles in the patient's care. The family provides emotional support, participates in shared decision making, performs much of the concrete caretaking, absorbs social and financial costs associated with the care of a dying family member, and works hard to maintain a sense of stability in the midst of change.[13] This list reveals how much the team depends on the family in achieving its own professional goals, and thus how important it is to maintain strong and positive relationships between the family and the team.

Second, when confronting expectations on the part of patients or family members that appear to conflict with the goals of palliative care, it is important to ask, *what are the origins of these expectations?* Are they, for example, indicators of patient or family denial, or have the patient and family been misled or confused by their care providers? Are seemingly inappropriate expectations the result of misunderstandings that are amenable to educational efforts, or signs of severe family stress or psychopathology that require more intensive psychological intervention?

Third, in the face of seemingly intractable conflict, there are often additional resources that can be brought to bear. For example, friends, other family members, or clergy can frequently play significant roles in resolving apparent impasses between family, patient, and team. In institutional settings, a hospital ethics committee can play a useful role in clarifying medical facts, permitting the ventilation of strong feelings, and exploring a wide range of options.

In summary, whatever the issue, setting, or combination of team members, family, and patient who are involved, open communication and mutual respect are the hallmarks of successful resolution of conflicting expectations in hospice and palliative care. This has been well expressed by Lederberg, who writes:

> When all is said and done, it cannot be overemphasized that the mainstay of management is the implementation of unhurried friendly discussions conducted in a spirit of open inquiry and genuine respect to encourage better communication between the principal parties.[14]

## ❖ Advance Directives

### *General Background*

There is now a strong societal and professional consensus in favor of patient self-determination in health care decision making, including decisions at the end of life. This consensus, which is reflected in legislation, judicial decisions, and official statements of professional societies and bioethics commissions, recognizes the right of competent adult patients to refuse or discontinue life-sustaining medical treatments.[15-19] While little controversy remains regarding the rights of competent patients who can communicate their preferences directly, extending these rights to patients who have lost decision-making capacity or who can no longer communicate continues to present difficulties.

Traditionally, health care decisions for nonautonomous patients have been made by physicians according to their best medical judgment, with varying degrees of consultation with the patient's family. Particularly since the 1960s, there has been growing concern that decisions made on this basis were leading to overtreatment of critically ill patients, subjecting them to prolonged dying in inappropriate, acute-care, high-technology settings. These same concerns were instrumental in the growth of the modern hospice movement. The answer to this problem was to give a greater role to the patient in these decisions, and to extend that role to the nonautonomous patient in the form of a written document containing his or her treatment preferences in the case of terminal illness.

Terms such as "advance directive," "living will," "health care proxy," and "durable power of attorney for health care" often are used interchangeably to refer to any document that is designed to permit a nonautonomous patient to direct his or her medical care at the end of life. Such documents are of two broad types. The first records the patient's specific preferences for treatment or nontreatment in various clinical situations. Treatments addressed most frequently are cardiopulmonary resuscitation, antibiotics for infection, blood transfusions, kidney dialysis, and artificial nutrition and hydration. The second type authorizes another person to speak for the nonautonomous patient at the time decisions actually have to be made. This document may or may not include the patient's specific preferences. Its chief virtue is that it empowers someone to make decisions on the patient's behalf on the basis of the actual medical circumstances that have arisen, rather than relying on preferences that the patient expressed in the past, when all of the medical circumstances were hypothetical.

In the United States, the public's awareness of the potential importance of advance directives was dramatically heightened by the publicity surrounding the case of Nancy Cruzan, a young woman whose parents had been prohibited by the Missouri Supreme Court from discontinuing lifesupports for her, even though she had been in a persistent vegetative state for seven years. The court's reasoning, which was upheld in 1990 by the U.S. Supreme Court, was that there was insufficient evidence that the parents' desire to discontinue treatment was in accord with what Nancy herself would have wanted.[20]

Also in 1990, the U.S. Congress passed the Patient Self-Determination Act. Effective since December 1, 1991, the PSDA requires health care institutions to inform all patients upon admission of their rights under state law to provide instructions regarding their medical treatment, their rights to refuse treatment, and their right to formulate advance directives.

Despite these influences, a growing body of empirical research has demonstrated that advance directives have had only a limited effect on health care decision making near the end of life. In part this is due to the small percentage of the population—ranging from a low of 10 percent to a high of 28 percent, the latter in a population of AIDS patients—that has formulated an advance directive. Even among patients who have them, a significant number of advance directives either fail to come to the attention of health care providers at the time decisions have to be made, are too vague to give meaningful guidance, or are disregarded on the grounds that the actual medical circumstances make the patient's stated preferences appear contrary to the patient's best interests at the time.[21,22]

Research on the effectiveness of advance directives and attempts to improve their acceptability and influence on decision making will certainly continue in the future. What is important about advance directives, however, is not the form itself, but the process of discussion and clarification of values that patients, families, and health professionals go through when the subject of advance directives is raised. Indeed, a better way to think of these issues is in terms of *advance planning*, rather than advance directives. The goal is for patients, families, and professionals—conferring and working together—to arrive at medical care decision making at the end of life that reflects the values and priorities of the patient. The process of enhancing patients' self-determination begins well before end-of-life decisions actually have to be made; it should be built into patient-provider communication at the inception of the caring relationship.[23]

This requires physicians, for example, to communicate openly and honestly with patients regarding the patient's medical condition and the likely outcomes of various therapeutic options. It requires patients to examine their own goals and values in light of what they know or can reasonably anticipate about their medical condition, and to decide how they would want decisions to be made should they lose their own decision-making capacity. In short, advance planning requires of both patients, families, and professionals the very candor and acknowledgment of the inevitability of physical decline and death that are hallmarks of hospice and palliative care.

## Advance Directives in Palliative Care

As Singer has pointed out, advance directives seem to be at once more and less relevant in the palliative care setting than elsewhere in health care.[24] They are more relevant because of the ubiquity of physical decline and death. They may be less relevant because patients who have elected to enter a hospice or palliative care setting are likely to have already decided to avoid many of the treatments which advance directives typically address.

As suggested earlier, however, there are still many decisions that have to be made within the hospice setting for which a clear sense of the patient's values and priorities is a critical ingredient in individualized decision making. Therefore, the broad guidelines for optimal advance planning and open communication mentioned in the previous section apply with equal force to hospice and palliative care, as well as in more active treatment settings. To say this is essentially to reinforce the earlier discussion of the importance of open communication in clarifying goals and expectations for hospice and palliative care at the outset, thereby minimizing conflicts of expectations among the patient, family members, and hospice team.

Moreover, there are a number of issues not directly related to *medical* decision making about which patients may have strong preferences, and which the team will want to know about in advance. These might include which friends and family members should be called as the patient's condition worsens, or special requests for prayers or other rituals near or after the time of death. Eliciting preferences such as these is clearly part of comprehensive palliative care, and the skills necessary to bring these matters into the open with patients and families are part of the necessary education for the hospice and palliative care professional.

## ❖ Physician-Assisted Suicide and Euthanasia

The subject of physician-assisted suicide and euthanasia has engaged philosophers, theologians, ethicists, health professionals, and policy makers for decades.[25-29] The current debate is taking place in the context of referenda and legislative proposals in several states that would change current law to permit physician-assisted suicide and/or active voluntary euthanasia. On November 8, 1994, the citizens of Oregon approved the Death with Dignity Act, the first of these proposals to be approved at the polls.[30] As this chapter was written, the Oregon law was under challenge in the courts and had not yet taken effect. What follows is a necessarily brief summary of the key issues in the debate, with special reference to its implications for hospice and palliative care.

### Definitions

Roy, Williams, and Dickens provide a clear and useful definition of euthanasia: "the deliberate, rapid, and painless termination of life of a person afflicted with incurable and progressive disease." What is usually referred to as "assisted suicide" they define as "assisted or self-administered euthanasia," that is, "when the sick person desiring to advance his or her death requires help from others, usually physicians or health care professionals, in obtaining lethal dosages of drugs and instructions on how to use these effectively."[31]

For the purposes of this discussion euthanasia and assisted suicide are both to be distinguished from two other medical actions: withholding or discontinuing life-sustaining treatment, and the administration of drugs for the relief of pain with the foreseeable but unintended side effect of hastening the dying process. These distinctions are themselves controversial. Some have argued that there is no moral difference between allowing a patient to die by withdrawing necessary life-supports, and acting with the deliberate intent to kill the patient. Both are deliberate actions that lead to the same result: The patient dies sooner than he or she otherwise would. To claim a moral difference between them, this argument runs, is to avoid facing up to the real issue that health professionals sometimes do kill their patients, but some acts of deliberate killing in medicine are justifiable.[25,32,33] In a similar vein, some would deny that a claimed difference in *intent* is sufficient to distinguish a lethal dose of pain medication, given for the relief of suffering, from an equivalent dose given to end the patient's life.[34]

Notwithstanding arguments such as these, the distinctions between withholding or withdrawing life-sustaining treatment and adequate pain control, on one side, and active euthanasia on the other, remain useful and valid both clinically and socially. They have been widely endorsed by professional organizations, bioethicists, and the courts.[17,31,35–40] In both cases, the issue of intent is crucial. In the case of withholding or withdrawing life-support, the primary intention is to refrain from useless or burdensome medical interventions that no longer benefit the patient. In the case of pain control, the intent is to relieve suffering with the appropriate use of medications. In neither case is the death of the patient the primary goal, as it unquestionably is in the case of active euthanasia or assisted suicide.

## ❖ The Paradigm Case and the Two Levels of Debate

The paradigm case for discussions of euthanasia and assisted suicide is that of a terminally ill patient who has concluded that his or her suffering—physical, psychological, or existential—is intolerable and beyond effective remedy, and who requests that he or she be helped to die, either by being given the knowledge and means to commit suicide, or by having his or her life ended quickly and painlessly through a lethal injection. The argument in favor of granting the patient's request rests on two main points: the patent's right to self-determination, and the obligation of health professionals to relieve suffering. An autonomous patient, who has concluded that his or her life is no longer of value to him or her because of extreme and irremediable suffering, ought to be able to choose the time and manner of his or her death. For a health professional to assist such a patient not only respects that patient's judgment regarding an acceptable quality of life, and his or her autonomy, but also acts beneficently in providing the patient relief from otherwise continuous suffering.

How should the hospice and palliative care team respond to such a request? The answer to this question involves considerations at two levels, which are closely intertwined but logically distinct. At the level of *direct clinical care* the question is: *Is it ever appropriate and morally justifiable for a health professional to respond affirmatively to the patient's request?* At the level of *public policy* the question is: *Even assuming that it is morally justifiable for a health professional to grant the patient's request, should our laws be changed so that it would be legal to do so?*

## Clinical Considerations

At the clinical level, the argument against granting the patient's request rests on the following main points. First, terminally ill patients who request help in hastening their deaths are frequently suffering from poorly controlled pain or other symptoms that are in fact amenable to effective palliative measures, or they are clinically depressed. Effective treatment of their symptoms or their depression usually results in the patient's repudiation of previously stated wishes to die.[41,42]

Second, the assumption that a patient who requests help in dying is truly autonomous is fallacious, not only because of the distorting effects of pain or depression, but also because dying patients are particularly vulnerable to feelings of worthlessness and of being a burden to others. These feelings make it likely that some patients' requests are not their own autonomous choices, but rather the choices they believe others want them to make.

Third, a patient's request for help in hastening death is often a way to express other things—loneliness, helplessness, fear—rather than a genuine wish for euthanasia. To take the request at face value without carefully probing its true significance for the patient would be a grievous error.

Thus, from the clinical standpoint, the appropriate and morally justifiable approach to a patient's request is to redouble efforts to identify the sources of the patient's suffering, and to apply palliative measures aggressively to alleviate them. This includes the full range of physical, psychological, and spiritual support.[41,43,44,45]

There are some who agree with the main thrust of these arguments and endorse aggressive palliative care as the appropriate clinical response to *most* patients' requests for assisted suicide or euthanasia, but nevertheless insist that there will always be two types of hard cases that urge us in the direction of complying with the patient's request. First, there are some patients whose pain or other symptoms are simply beyond effective palliative measures. Second, there are patients whose main source of suffering is not physical but existential: Life has simply become a torment and an intolerable burden to them for reasons that are rooted in their own deeply held, individual values. The authors of this book argue not only that granting these patients' requests is morally and clinically justifiable, but also that public policy should be changed so that such acts on the part of physicians would be legal.[46,47]

There is, however, one more option that can be offered to these patients: continuous sedation.[48] The preference for continuous sedation over active euthanasia in these cases of extreme and otherwise irremediable suffering is based primarily on the broader public policy implications of professional or societal sanction of euthanasia.

## Public Policy Considerations

To those who believe that physician-assisted suicide and active voluntary euthanasia are sometimes morally valid and appropriate clinical responses, the distinction between continuous sedation and euthanasia seems vanishingly thin, if not hypocritical. And yet, in those rare cases where effective palliative measures are either lacking or are rejected by the patient, to offer sedation rather than to legalize euthanasia or physician-assisted suicide is the best social policy. Why?

The overriding concern with the legalization of physician-assisted suicide or active euthanasia is the possibility of abuses. The major disagreement between advocates and opponents of changes in current law is over the nature and likelihood of potential abuses of a more permissive policy, and the reliability of various safeguards that have been proposed to prevent them.

Every plausible proposal for a change in the law restricts physician-assisted suicide and active euthanasia to the competent patient, suffering irremediably from a documented terminal illness, who makes repeated requests over time. Various safeguards, such as confirmation of diagnosis and prognosis, psychiatric examinations, and documented offers of "state-of-the-art" palliative care, are proposed to prevent premature compliance with such a request, or the expansion of the policy to include patients for whom assisted suicide or euthanasia would be nonvoluntary or even involuntary. Were such a policy adopted, however, there are several reasons to worry that the initial scope of the practice of assisted suicide and active euthanasia would in time expand beyond the original intent of the law.

First, recall that the foundations of the argument to adopt a more permissive policy are the values of *self-determination* and *relief of suffering*. The logic of the value of self-determination dictates that restricting the law to patients with a "terminal illness" is highly arbitrary. Who defines when a patient is "terminal," and therefore eligible for assisted suicide or euthanasia? Why shouldn't the patient—according to the value of self-determination—be able to preempt the suffering entailed in a long, progressive illness, and choose the time and manner of his of her death regardless of the timing of that decision? Similarly, if the motivation for the new law is the relief of suffering, why restrict its scope to the suffering that is due to a terminal illness? Why should it not be up to the individual to determine that his or her life is no longer of value, for reasons peculiar to him or herself?

A second reason to anticipate the eventual expansion of the practices envisioned in a new law derives from the history of the movement to allow patients to refuse life-support. Initially only a competent, terminally ill patient was allowed to do this. But it was soon convincingly argued that a person should not lose the right to decline burdensome life-supporting medical care simply because he or she had ceased to be competent or autonomous. Hence, as described above, advance directives and surrogate decision makers have been incorporated into policy and law to extend the right to refuse medical care to nonautonomous patients. There is no reason to suppose that a similar expansion of the "right" to assisted suicide and active euthanasia will not be similarly enacted, should an initially more restrictive policy be adopted.

Finally, the safeguards related to ruling out mental illness and other attestations of the patient's genuine autonomy may be illusory in practice. The aged and dying occupy vulnerable places in the social fabric as it is. Financial pressures, generational conflicts, the stigma attached to certain diseases such as AIDS, the enormous stresses associated with efforts to care for a dying family member at home, and the very uneven access to excellent palliative care, combine to create a societal context in which it is quite plausible to expect significant abuses of a more permissive policy for "voluntary" assisted suicide or euthanasia.

In this context, neither physician-assisted suicide nor active euthanasia should be legalized. It is correct, as advocates of a change in current law argue, that maintaining current prohibitions against these practices is an abridgement of personal liberty. But such an abridgement is justified in light of the potential abuses and harms that could plausibly follow a new policy. Furthermore, the expansion of excellent palliative care services, which are severely underfunded and unevenly available to the population as a whole, can reduce even further the already small number of patients for whom assisted suicide or euthanasia are truly the only desirable options. Even the most articulate and forceful advocates of new laws which would permit physician-assisted suicide and euthanasia, recommend the expansion of palliative care services.[49] In the context of the very real need for palliative care, as well as the pressures for new and potentially dangerous social policies, the improvement and expansion of palliative care are important social goals. Advocacy for these improvements, and not for more permissive policies for assisted suicide and euthanasia, is the proper ethical course for health professionals.

## ❖ Summary

This chapter has discussed several ethical issues commonly encountered in hospice and palliative care: conflicting expectations of patients, families, and the hospice team; communication about diagnosis and prognosis; pain management; advance directives and decision making for the nonautonomous patient; and physician-assisted suicide and euthanasia. A common thread linking all of these issues is the importance of clear, sensitive communication with patients and families that respects the uniqueness of the individual. From its inception, the caring relationship should be characterized by open communication, the provision of accurate and realistic information, and clarification of values and preferences. This approach offers the best hope of avoiding serious ethical conflicts, and provides the foundation of trust and open communication necessary to resolve conflicts that do arise.

Clear, sensitive communication is especially important when patients' extreme suffering prompts requests for assisted suicide or euthanasia. The team must make every effort to understand the specific nature of the patient's suffering, and to provide the appropriate physical, psychological, or spiritual support, which may require attending to the needs of the patient's family as well. In the rare cases where palliative measures fail or are rejected by the patient, continuous sedation, and not compliance with the patient's request, is the morally preferable alternative. Though refusing the patient's request appears to be an abridgment of personal liberty, it is justified in order to prevent the abuses that could very plausibly follow a more permissive social policy.

## ❖ References

1. Buckman, R. *How to Break Bad News: A Guide for Health Professionals.* Toronto: University of Toronto Press, 1992.
2. Weisman, A. "The Patient with a Fatal Illness: To Tell or Not to Tell." *Journal of the American Medical Association,* 201:646–648, 1967.
3. Fitch, M.I. "How Much Should I Say to Whom?" *Journal of Palliative Care,* 10(3):90–100, 1994.
4. Bowen, M. "Family Reaction to Death." In Philip J. Guerin, Jr., ed. *Family Therapy: Theory and Practice.* New York: Gardner Press, 1976.
5. Northouse, P.G., and Northouse, L.L. "Communication and Cancer: Issues Confronting Patients, Health Professionals, and Family Members." *Journal of Psychosocial Oncology,* 5(3):17–46, 1987.
6. Vachon, M.L.S. "Emotional Problems in Palliative Care: Patient, Family, and Professional." In D. Doyle, G.W.C. Hanks, N. MacDonald, eds. *Oxford Textbook of Palliative Medicine.* Oxford: Oxford University Press, 1993.
7. Weisman, A. *On Dying and Denying: A Psychiatric Study of Terminality.* New York: Behavioral Publications, 1972.
8. Wool, M.S. "Understanding Denial in Cancer Patients." *Advances in Psychosomatic Medicine,* 18:35–53, 1988.
9. Psychological Work Group of the International Work Group on Death, Dying, and Bereavement. "A Statement of Assumptions and Principles Concerning Psychological Care of Dying Persons and Their Families." *Journal of Palliative Care,* 9(3):29–32, 1993.
10. Jacox, A.K., et al. *Management of Cancer Pain: Clinical Practice Guideline.* No. 9 AHCPR Publication No. 94-0592. Rockville, MD: Agency for Health Care Policy and Research, 1994.
11. Burge, F.I. "I Would Never Do That!" *Journal of Palliative Care,* 10(3):73–75, 1994.
12. Henteleff, P.D. "We Don't Do That in Palliative Care." *Journal of Palliative Care,* 10(3):76–78, 1994.
13. Rait, D., and Lederberg, M. "The Family of the Cancer Patient." In J.C. Holland and J.H. Rowland, eds. *Handbook of Psychooncology.* New York: Oxford University Press, 1990.
14. Lederberg, M. "The Confluence of Psychiatry, the Law and Ethics." In J.C. Holland and J.H. Rowland, eds. *Handbook of Psychooncology.* New York: Oxford University Press, 1990.

15. ACCP/SCCM Consensus Panel. "Ethical and Moral Guidelines for the Initiation, Continuation, and Withdrawal of Intensive Care." *Chest, 97*:949–958, 1990.

16. American Thoracic Society. "Withholding and Withdrawing Life-Sustaining Therapy." *Annals of Internal Medicine, 115*:478–485, 1991.

17. Council on Ethical and Judicial Affairs, American Medical Association. "Decisions Near the End of Life." *Journal of the American Medical Association, 267*:2229–2233, 1992.

18. Gostin, L.O., and Weir, R. "Life and Death Choices after Cruzan: Case Law and Standards of Professional Conduct." *Milbank Quarterly, 64*:143–173, 1991.

19. The Hastings Center. *Guidelines on the Termination of Life-Sustaining Treatment and the Care of the Dying.* Briarcliff Manor, NY: The Hastings Center, 1987.

20. *Cruzan v Director.* Missouri Department of Health, 110 S.CT 2841, 1990.

21. Teno, J.M., et al. "Do Formal Advance Directives Affect Resuscitation Decisions and the Use of Resources for Seriously Ill Patients?" *Journal of Clinical Ethics, 5*(1):23–30, 1994.

22. Danis, M., et al. "A Prospective Study of Advance Directives for Life-Sustaining Care." *New England Journal of Medicine, 324*:882–887, 1991.

23. Barnard, D. "Advance Directives." In R.C. Bone, et al., eds. *Pulmonary and Critical Care Medicine.* St. Louis: Mosby–Year Book, 1994.

24. Singer, P.A. "Advance Directives in Palliative Care." *Journal of Palliative Care 10*(3):111–116, 1994.

25. Brock, D. "Voluntary Active Euthanasia." *The Hastings Center Report, 22*(2):10–22, 1992.

26. Kamisar, Y. "Some Non-religious Views against Proposed 'Mercy Killing' Legislation." *Minnesota Law Review, 42*(6):969–1042, 1958.

27. Quill, T. "Death and Dignity: A Case of Individualized Decision Making." *New England Journal of Medicine, 327*:691–694, 1991.

28. Singer, P.A., and Siegler, M. "Euthanasia—A Critique." *New England Journal of Medicine, 322*:1881–1883, 1990.

29. Weir, R. "The Morality of Physician-assisted Suicide." *Law, Medicine, and Health Care, 20*(1–2):116–126, 1992.

30. Oregon State Legislature, Measure Number 16: *Death with Dignity Act.* November 8, 1994.

31. Roy, D.J., et al. *Bioethics in Canada.* Ontario: Prentice Hall Canada, 1994, 411–412.

32. Rachels, J. "Active and Passive Euthanasia." *New England Journal of Medicine, 292*:78–80, 1975.

33. Brody, H. "Causing, Intending, and Assisting Death." *Journal of Clinical Ethics, 4*(2):112–117, 1993.

34. Quill, T. "The Ambiguity of Clinical Intentions." *New England Journal of Medicine, 329*:1039–1040, 1993.

35. American College of Physicians Health and Public Policy Committee. "Drug Therapy for Severe Chronic Pain in Terminal Illness." *Annals of Internal Medicine, 99*:870–880, 1983.

36. American Pain Society. *Principles of Analgesic Use in the Treatment of Acute Pain and Chronic Cancer Pain,* 4th ed. Skokie, IL: American Pain Society, 1992.

37. World Health Organization. *Cancer Pain Relief and Palliative Care.* Geneva: World Health Organization, 1990.

38. Spross, J.A., et al. "Oncology Nursing Society Position Paper on Cancer Pain Part I." *Oncology Nursing Forum, 17*(4):595–614, 1990.

39. Spross, J.A., et al. "Oncology Nursing Society Position Paper on Cancer Pain, Part II." *Oncology Nursing Forum, 17*(5):751–760, 1990.

40. Gostin, L.O. "Drawing a Line between Killing and Letting Die: The Law, the Law Reform, on Medically Assisted Dying." *The Journal of Law, Medicine, and Ethics, 21*(1):94–101, 1993.

41. Foley, K.M. "The Relationship of Pain and Symptom Management to Patient Requests for Physician-assisted Suicide." *Journal of Pain and Symptom Management, 6*(5):289–297, 1991.

42. Breitbart, W. "Suicide." In J.C. Holland and J.H. Rowland, eds. *Handbook of Psychooncology.* New York: Oxford University Press, 1990.

43. Byock, I.R. "Consciously Walking the Fine Line: Thoughts on a Hospice Response to Assisted Suicide and Euthanasia." *Journal of Palliative Care, 9*(3):25–28, 1993.

44. Moulin, D.E., et al. "Statement on Euthanasia and Physician-assisted Suicide." *Journal of Palliative Care, 10*(2):80–81, 1994.

45. Saunders, C. "Voluntary Euthanasia." *Palliative Medicine, 6*(1):1–5, 1992.

46. Quill, T. *Death and Dignity: Making Choices and Taking Charge.* New York: Norton, 1993.

47. Brody, H. "Assisted Death: A Compassionate Response to a Medical Failure." *New England Journal of Medicine, 327:*1384–1388, 1992.

48. Cherny, N.I., and Portenoy, R.K. "Sedation in the Management of Refractory Symptoms: Guidelines for Evaluation and Treatment." *Journal of Palliative Care, 10*(2):31–38, 1994.

49. Miller, F.G., et al. "Regulating Physician-assisted Death." *New England Journal of Medicine, 331:*119–123, 1994.

# ❖ Chapter 13

# Support Groups for Hospice Staff

Leonard J. Zamborsky

Stress might be likened to a violin string: Stretched to the appropriate length, the violin string does its work of providing music. A lack of tension will mean no music, while too much tension will cause the string to break. Stress is a necessary part of life. Healthy stress encourages efficiency and excellence in the use of time and resources. Unhealthy or disproportionate stress can cause individual or organizational breakdown.

## ❖ Stress Specific to Hospice Work

Hospice staff are confronted on a day-to-day basis with human situations that are emotionally draining. Terminally ill people and their families are confronted with grief. In addition, the dynamics of the family system enter into the process and directly affect the hospice worker. Families that are basically healthy bring the resources and strength of the family unit to the situation of dealing with a dying loved one. Families that have significant "unfinished business" or unresolved conflicts may not have the necessary strength to deal with this stressful life event. The hospice worker experiences a range of emotions in the psychodynamics of the terminally ill person and the family system.[1]

The hospice worker's professional or paraprofessional training, emphasising professional and ethical standards while providing guidelines that can make decisions easier, also increases stress. One of the strengths of hospice care is that it is holistic in response to the terminally ill person and family and is based on an interdisciplinary approach with strong team models. While the team's holistic, interdisciplinary approach is meant to share the load, it may increase the demands and stress placed upon the team as a whole and individual members.[2,3] Mutual respect, cooperative action, and good communication are the hallmarks of an effective team. All of this takes effort and expends energy.

Other sources of stress include the hospice workers' own human situations, intrapersonal psychodynamics, and the usually late arrival in the course of the terminal illness with little history or familiarity with the individual and family. The hospice worker is expected to be able to intercede in the complex intense emotional and personal issues during this time of potential crisis. In working with the terminally ill and their families, one also confronts one's own mortality and personal relationships.[1] Even the healthiest and most balanced individual, when challenged with caring for someone their own age, with the same number of children, and with a very similar marital relationship, may experience additional stress.

As the hospice movement has become more well known, demands for hospice care have grown. The larger case loads, rapid turnover, high patient acuity, and working in many different home settings rather than in the traditional structured hospital setting where the professional was trained and empowered, increase the stress on hospice workers.[1]

### ❖ The Value of a Support Group

Hospice staff who are able to face their own feelings and issues and work them through in an appropriate way will be able to continue their work with a high degree of competency, and with an equally high degree of human compassion. Participating in a staff support group is one way to cope with the stress specific to hospice work—one way to keep the violin tuned.[2,4,5] A support group is a self assistance group, which is professionally facilitated. Hospice provides holistic quality care to individuals with life threatening illnesses and their families. A hospice staff support group provides the opportunity to discuss feelings and work through emotional issues in a safe environment.

People who work in situations that are emotionally demanding often find that their loved ones are not able to give them the level and kind of support they need. It is fairly typical of a loved one to offer solutions or to try to "fix" things in other ways. It is much more helpful for individuals to express their feelings. The support group supplies a qualitatively different kind of assistance that allows this expression.[6] Support group members understand in a different way because they share in the work with its challenges and satisfactions. One of the benefits of a support group is that members know they are not alone. Others share similar feelings and experiences.

The support group is a safe place for people to be aware of their feelings and to express them, to listen to the information that feelings offer, and to clarify choices. In this way, the support group is an antidote to burnout and can help individuals remain in good health and balance.[1] Coming to the group to both support others and be supported is an appropriate technique for hospice workers to handle stress.

### ❖ Norms for Support Groups

Confidentiality among members is extremely important. In situations where confidentiality is broken, directly or indirectly, not only does the support group malfunction, it becomes a source of great stress and potentially great harm. Confidentiality creates a safe environment for self expression. It means that what happens in the group stays in the group. What is expressed or experienced in the group is neither repeated outside the group nor discussed by some of the group outside the group time. If a group member feels a need to address anything about the group or a group member, the agreement to confidentiality means that the subject will be brought up with the entire group or discussed privately and professionally with the facilitator.

Some individuals want to set an issue or feeling aside once they have said what they need to during group and once they have heard supportive responses. While it may be appropriate to offer a colleague a word or gesture of support outside group time, caution is necessary. The group member needs to judge whether or not such expressions would be wanted or helpful.

A nonjudgmental acceptance of each other's feelings and perceptions is also necessary if members are going to feel free to express themselves. While individuals perceive, experience, and handle things differently, it is crucial that group members accept each other. When someone does not agree with the choice or decision of another group member, it is helpful to express acceptance of the person before offering any feedback. Support group serves a completely different function from case review or supervision. The "no advice" rule is a consequence of nonjudgmental acceptance and the fact that support group is not a problem-solving meeting. Responses that indicate what one should or should not do or feel will be a major inhibitor to effective support and sharing. It can be beneficial, however, for members to talk about what has been helpful to them in similar situations.

A mutual commitment to be present is important to the individual and the group. Members often say they are glad they came to support group on the very day it was most difficult. Moreover, members are never totally aware of what their presence or absence can mean to others. Someone, for example, may perceive another's absence as a reaction to what was said during the previous meeting. An individual's absence may also include the absence of the necessary support for another's sharing. It is helpful, therefore, for group members to agree that if an emergency or serious situation arises that will keep them from coming, they will inform the group through one of the members. Support group is a safe place to cope with stress because it provides for the specific needs of the group. These are outlined in Table 13–1.

TABLE 13–1   Elements Provided by a Support Group to Make It a Safe Place to Cope with Stress

Confidentiality

Nonjudgmental acceptance by the participants

A "no advice" rule

Commitment by the participants to be present

Mutual responsibility among participants

Benefits for all the participants

Mutual responsibility is also essential for the group. Each member agrees to let the group know what is wanted, liked, or disliked and respects the right or need of others to group time. While at times one or another member may utilize more of the group time, sensitivity to balance is required. This commitment implies an understanding that the support group exists for the benefit of all. Support group is not a "complaint department." Problems, issues, and situations that need to be dealt with by supervisors or management personnel are not the subject matter of support group. It is appropriate for group members to express feelings related to the organization and difficulties in the working environment. Others may acknowledge that they share similar feelings or experiences, and encouragement to effectively resolve difficulties is shared.

### ❖ Role of the Facilitator

The director of Human Resources may hire and supervise the work of competent facilitators for support groups. The body of knowledge and training experiences included in the preparation of professionals in the field of group work provide the required background for a support group facilitator. Usually, therefore, the facilitator would be a psychologist or a similarly prepared professional who is hired as a consultant.

In their training, facilitators will have learned about the dynamics of group interaction, the course of group development, the procedures that enable positive movement, the necessary and appropriate interventions, and the ethical imperatives inherent in group work. The following is not an effort to comprehensively or exhaustively discuss the group facilitator's role or procedures. It is an enumeration of dimensions of the facilitating role.

The facilitator clarifies group norms, procedures, and or "rules" before or during the initial group session. When the need arises, the facilitator reminds individuals or the group about the norms. At times, this maintaining of norms will include further explanation or elaboration. Attending to the need for all members to have group time, the facilitator responds both to individuals who have a tendency to monopolize and to those that have a tendency to be silent.

At the very heart of the facilitating role is the awareness of the process that is taking place along with the layers of intrapersonal and interpersonal psychodynamics. Using their acquired skills, facilitators support the movement of the group in a helpful direction frequently by making the group aware of the current dynamics of the process. They also pay special attention to individual and collective cues relative to content and themes. When themes emerge which the group agrees to focus on, the facilitator invites the group to express their feelings and awarenesses.

It is within the competency and professional responsibility of the facilitator both to recognize individual needs and to intervene appropriately. Most often this responsibility can be executed by the facilitator spending a few moments after the group meeting to share awareness with the individual and to offer possibilities and suggestions for healthy resolution of inner conflicts. After the group meeting, for example, the facilitator might discuss with an individual possible resolutions of "unfinished business" with a parent. A more striking example would be the situation in which the facilitator recognizes standard and significant signs of serious depression.

## ❖ Group Membership and Methodology

Wherever hospice organizations are able to implement support groups, the ideal is to offer this benefit to every employee. Along with clinical staff, the office staff share in some of the stress related to this kind of work. Ideally, the support group is offered both as an acknowledgment of the stress specific to hospice work, and as a cost-effective, compassionate means of maintaining a stable and healthy staff who continue to experience joy, satisfaction, and meaning in their hospice work. The budget would, therefore, include reimbursement for a facilitator.[7]

Management of the hospice organization provides adequate space and time during the working day for support groups as well as coverage for the responsibilities of the group members.[7] If a hospice employee attends an hour-and-a-half support group meeting in addition to the usual number of daily visits or other responsibilities, the support group meeting itself becomes a source of further stress and pressure.

There are many possible configurations for hospice staff support groups. One workable pattern might be to provide 10 one-and-a-half hour sessions for eight to ten participants. The sessions would be scheduled at convenient times on a biweekly basis. A few weeks after the twenty-week sequence has been completed, another ten-session segment would begin. Every time a new sequence begins, staff members would have the opportunity to sign up for support group. Near the end of the twenty weeks, the group individually and collectively evaluates the effectiveness. Modifications in terms of scheduling, methodology, and facilitators are undertaken. The length of time, the number of participants, the scheduling, and other parameters of the group are determined by the desire to maximize the benefits within the confines of resources. Individual sessions usually have a pattern which either is outlined and agreed upon at the beginning or emerges over time (Table 13–2). A helpful pattern which allows the facilitator and all members to be aware of individual and collective needs and issues begins with a "check-in" on the part of each member. This consists of going around the circle to provide each member an opportunity to express feelings and briefly state issues or concerns they may wish to address. The habit of identifying and expressing one's feelings is itself a helpful and healthy antidote to the effects of stress. The facilitator can determine the amount of time to spend with an individual or on a specific topic. At times the group will agree to focus on an emergent theme.

TABLE 13–2   Common Techniques Used in Support Groups

Checking in

Sharing feelings and experiences

Receiving feedback

Discussing topics

Telling stories

Using art, music, and visual imagery

A variety of group approaches and activities are employed to benefit the group. Sharing feelings and experiences and receiving feedback about what individuals have found helpful often takes place. Genuine and accepting response are at the very heart of the therapeutic effect of group participation. Discussions of topics of common interest is another common activity. Telling stories about patients and family members facilitates the grief work necessary for staff members.

Music, art, movement, and other forms of expressive therapy are also quite helpful. In the receptive mode, group members look at art, observe movement, or listen to music that can help express feelings or experience relaxation. Through expressive approaches, participants can deal with and work through dimensions of their feelings or conflicts that they may not have been aware of. In one example, the facilitator uses a soft clear voice uttered with a soothing rhythm and cadence which matches background music of nature or human artistry. Group members are invited to imagine themselves sitting in the woods with their feet in a stream, dropping their burdens on leaves that flow rapidly out of sight. In another case, the participants respond to the invitation to pick any color and to begin to apply it to the paper without any conscious or rational thought. Members begin to express feelings of anger or peace, pain, or confusion. The artistic adventure has itself allowed some feelings to be expressed, and the personal analysis or discussion often leads to new levels of awareness and discovery.

A variety of relaxation techniques can be helpful to individuals and the whole group. Relaxation breathing, deep muscle relaxation, fantasy, and imagining can be used individually or collectively to help relieve stress or perhaps to make contact with ultimate reality. Relaxation approaches are often combined with expressive approaches for a more holistic benefit.

## ❖ Summary

Hospice support groups provide an opportunity for staff to cope with the stresses associated with hospice work. This is one way for the hospice management to validate the stresses associated with hospice work and offer support from the organization. A safe environment and competent facilitator are integral components to an effective group. The techniques used during the group session may be as varied as the participants.

## ❖ References

1. Ray, E., Nichols, M.R., and Perritt, L.J. "A Model of Job Stress and Burnout." *Hospice Journal*, 3(2–3):3–28, 1987.
2. Schneider, J. "Self-care: Challenges and Rewards for Hospice Professionals." *Hospice Journal*, 3(2–3):255–276, 1987.
3. Vachon, M. *Occupational Stress in the Case of the Critically Ill, the Dying and the Bereaved*. Bristol, PA: Hemisphere Publishers, 1987.
4. Parry, J.K. "Mutual Support for Hospice Staff: Planned or Ad Hoc?" *Journal of Palliative Care*, 5(1):34–36, 1989.
5. Parry, J.K. "Mutual Support Groups: Do They Relieve Staff Stress?" *Jewish Social Work Forum*, 25:43–49, 1989.
6. Larson, D.G. *The Helper's Journey: Working with People Facing Grief, Loss, and Life-threatening Illness*. Champaign, IL: Research Press, 1993.
7. Richman, J.M. "Groupwork in a Hospice Setting." *Social Work with Groups*, 12(4):171–184, 1989.

## ❖ For Further Reading

Finlay, I. "Sources of Stress in Hospice Medical Directors and Matrons." *Palliative Medicine*, 4:5–9, 1989.

Glass, J., Conrad, J., and Hastings, J.L. "Stress and Burnout: Concerns for the Hospice Volunteer." *Educational-Gerontology*, 18:715–731, 1992.

Harris, R.D., Bond, M.J., and Turnbull, R. "Nursing Stress and Stress Reduction in Palliative Care." *Palliative Medicine*, 4:191–196, 1990.

Larson, D.G. "Developing Effective Hospice Staff Support Groups: Pilot Test of an Innovative Training Program." *Hospice Journal*, 2(2):41–55, 1986.

Larson, D.G. "Helper Secrets: Invisible Stressors in Hospice Work." *American Journal of Hospice Care*, 35–40, November/December, 1985.

Masterson, A., et al. "Staff Burnout in a Hospice Setting." *Hospice Journal*, 1(3):1–15, 1985.

Patrick, P.K. "Hospice Caregiving: Strategies to Avoid Burnout and Maintain Self-preservation." *Hospice Journal*, 3(2–3):223–253, 1987.

Vachon, M. "Myths and Realities in Palliative/Hospice Care." *Hospice Journal*, 2(1):63–79, 1986.

# ❖ Chapter 14

# Inclusion in American Health Care

John J. Mahoney

In the 1982 best seller *Megatrends,* author John Naisbitt identified the hospice movement as part of the "ten new directions transforming our lives." Specifically, Naisbitt credited the anticipated growth of hospice care as a response to technology, the now famous, "high tech/high touch" formula. He also wrote that hospice care would benefit from his so-called sixth new direction—the movement from institutional help to "self-help."[1]

Although few knew it then, Naisbitt was forecasting the direction of our society, particularly as it relates to health care, in a relatively stable period of growth. Certainly no one ten years ago was able to predict the direction health care is now taking, nor the pace of change. Predicting the next ten years of health care evolution and how hospice care and programs will fit into that changing environment will not be easy, and comes with no guarantees.

Although his book was remarkably accurate as to the growing success of hospice care in the United States, the hospice movement Naisbitt wrote about in 1982 only remotely resembles hospice care of today.

## ❖ Hospice Beginnings

From the first hospice program in 1974 and prior to 1982, hospice programs existed solely on grants, community donations, and small fees for service plans. In 1982, the Medicare hospice benefit was enacted into law, and the funding of hospice programs began to stabilize as hospice care began to be more widely acknowledged by other health care providers and payers. Interestingly, this acknowledgement by health care insurers of the benefits of hospice care was not initially well received by everyone in the hospice movement, and the ensuing struggle and conflict around the development of a comprehensive standard of services that would be hospice care as we know it today under Medicare almost destroyed the hospice movement as it grappled with the issues of reimbursement, government oversight, and public scrutiny.

In 1982, the hospice movement was guided by women and men who saw the need to provide compassionate care to terminally ill individuals caught up in a system that was increasingly impersonal and neglectful of their needs—their need for adequate pain and symptom control; their need to have the dignity they had cherished all their lives be even more highly respected at the end of their lives; their need to be embraced by their caregiver as a living person, and not to be considered as just the sum of their collective symptoms; and their need to continue to feel part of their family community and their friends community, and not to be isolated from either.

The enthusiasm for hospice care at the time was borne out of knowledge that what hospice was doing was addressing not only the patient's suffering, but also the suffering of the patient's family. Hospice understood that what it provided was more than medical care, that in a comprehensive case-managed manner it was bringing to patient and family, for the first time, a philosophy of care that addressed the physical, spiritual, and psychosocial needs of the patient and family. These were the keys to the unique nature of hospice care in 1974 and 1982. Almost two decades later, no other form of care offers this type of service.

Successful though it was, hospice was not without serious limitations. Hospice programs were not particularly well managed. Hospice proponents considered hospice care as an alternative to traditional health care and saw themselves rejecting "form" in favor of "substance." Access to hospice care was severely limited. Hospice programs were increasingly successful caring for cancer patients, and although the care being provided was of very high quality, it depended greatly on the fact that the complexity of the patients hospices served was limited.

## ❖ Hospice Today

In the introduction to his book, Naisbitt notes that the most reliable way to anticipate the future is by understanding the present.[1] The National Hospice Organization estimates that currently 340,000 patients are being served each year by approximately 2,500 hospices in the United States. Both statistics have more than doubled in the last ten years. While certainly impressive, such numbers also illustrate the limits of predicting the future. In 1985, NHO predicted that in 1995 there would be as many as 6,800 hospices in the United States.

Hospices today are still relatively small providers. Hospices have an average annual census of approximately 120 to 130 patients per year. However, the median program is increasing in size, which illustrates one possible future trend—the number of hospices in the future will not increase with the same level of growth, and many of the existing programs will grow much larger.

The organizational structure of hospice care has remained relatively stable over the years, with approximately 40 percent being independent programs, 30 percent being hospital based, 24 percent home health based, and the remainder having various organizational structures such as government based or nursing home based.[2]

Of the $200 plus billion of the 1993 Medicare expenditures, hospice care represents approximately $1 billion, and perhaps as much as $1.5 billion of the total national health care bill, estimated at more than $1 trillion. While perhaps not startling as a percentage of health care funding, a billion dollars is a tremendous amount of money when one thinks about the humble origins of this movement. To put it into perspective, the *1994 Green Book* (The Committee on Ways and Means U.S. House of Representatives Overview of Entitlement Programs) reports that Medicare spent more than $3.5 billion in 1992 on eye-related surgical specialists.

## ❖ Trends in Hospice Care

Hospices continue to serve primarily cancer patients. However, programs are beginning to serve individuals with other illnesses in greater numbers. Hospices serve approximately 35 percent of people who die of cancer as well as approximately 35 percent of people who die of AIDS. Nationally, hospices have begun to serve minority communities in more representative numbers. The efforts of the National Hospice Organization and the chair of its task force on access to hospice care by minorities, Bernice Catherine Harper, have been instrumental in this work.

While Naisbitt's predictions were made in the midst of relative stability, they are remarkable nonetheless. However, predicting the future of hospice care today gives new meaning to the term "challenge." Still, like Naisbitt we can examine trends and current indicators to achieve a certain clarity in the crystal ball.

As the chapter for this book was being written in the fall of 1994, there were several trends developing simultaneously that will have significant impact on both hospice care and the programs that deliver that care at the bedside of the terminally ill. First, even though the Congress of the United States failed to adopt a major health care reform package, it is probable that the 104th Congress will consider a modest package of reforms that could include restructuring the Medicaid system.

Regardless of activity at the national level, health care reform has already begun and will accelerate because policy changes are also taking place at the same level. In his book, Naisbitt identified several states as being on the cutting edge of innovation, including California, Florida, Washington, Colorado, and Connecticut. From a hospice perspective, it is difficult to argue with that designation. Connecticut was the site of the first hospice in the United States, followed closely by hospices in California, Florida, and Colorado. It is also well known that the leadership of the hospice movement in the past 20 years has drawn heavily from the ranks of hospice programs in those states.

Again Florida, Colorado, and Washington are among those states leading reform efforts at the state level. States have reached a point where they no longer feel capable of containing their Medicaid costs. The Governors estimate that 25 percent of their budgets will shortly be consumed by Medicaid, and these three states, joined by others such as Oregon and Tennessee, are leading the effort to reverse that trend. These efforts primarily rely on the state receiving waivers from the federal government from certain Medicaid requirements, and greater reliance on managed care companies.

Perhaps most importantly, the American business community has taken an increasing activist role in the management and delivery of health care to their employees. This "downward" pressure from the payers of health insurance premiums and users of health care has forced providers and insurers to seek creative alternatives to a system of health care delivery that cannot even be characterized as the "current" system, as it is already in great flux.

These trends will continue, and the hospice movement will have little direct impact on the direction of these trends. Health care providers are not driving this reform—they are responding to it as seen in the creation of new provider and insurance coalitions through alliances, mergers, and acquisitions. The health care environment is moving inevitably toward a system that will increasingly reward so-called managed care networks, limiting the opportunity for success of individual providers, whether they are hospitals, home health agencies, doctors, or hospices unless they participate in these newly developing coalitions.

These forces will result in increased competition among insurers and between providers—including hospices as they all seek to maintain their market share. Additionally, all providers will be required to give greater services at reduced reimbursement. It is highly likely that the quality of health care services will decline in the short term as the states and new systems struggle with issues of eligibility, coverage, standards of care, and practice guidelines.

Additionally, a great deal of emphasis has been placed on the positive aspects of the informed consumer forcing providers and insurers to offer a quality product and provide quality services; however, the measurements necessary to provide the information we need as consumers, in a form that less sophisticated consumers will be able to comprehend and use in their decision making, is still many years away from being readily available. As these measurements become more widely available, the quality of care will improve again as the market and reimbursement stabilize and consumers begin to have the information necessary to demand the quality of services they deserve.

As competition increases it is likely that there will be fewer hospices in some cities and regions as hospices go out of business or merge. This will be particularly true where we have multiple hospices in moderate-sized cities. Those hospices that will remain will, on average, be larger in the long term than they are today. Additionally, it is likely that more of the hospice programs in the future will be for-profit enterprises. This will result from increasing difficulty of receiving a charitable designation from the IRS simply because of an organization's status as a health care provider.

## ❖ Looking into the Future of Hospice

The immediate future for hospice care, that is, the next three years, is relatively well assured. The immediate future for hospice programs themselves will be marked more by rough seas than calm waters. However, hospices are not strictly at the mercy of the winds of change. There are initiatives and innovations that hospice programs can embark upon to not only increase their chances of survival, but actually enhance their thriving in these most extraordinary times.

First, the Board of Directors of each hospice must understand the dynamics and speed of this changing marketplace environment, and they have to integrate that knowledge into their strategic planning. Using a phrase from noted management guru and author Tom Peter, hospices will need to be ready to "abandon," not just reformat some of their current thinking, structure, and services.[3]

Second, the Chief Executive Officers (CEO) of hospices of the future will need to be exceptional managers. The changing environment of health care will be nothing less than chaotic over the next few years. How well hospice managers respond to managing in such an ambiguous marketplace will determine in great measure how successful they will be as individuals, and how well the hospice program functions going into the next decade. It is important to understand that the reference here is not to just managing change—nothing is static. Managing "change" is a continuous process, but it does not describe the turmoil health care, including hospice care, will experience over the next few years. The successful manager will understand and demonstrate what Peter Drucker, a well-known businessman and author, identifies as the ability to manage situations where the manager is neither in control nor is the manager being controlled.[4] The standard of evaluation will not be how many people one manages or even the size of the budget, but how successfully one manages the complexities of the job, the information it uses and generates, and the relationships needed to do the work of the organization.[4]

Of particular importance will be those relationships with other providers and insurers in the development of networks and alliances. Providers participating in networks to create "one-stop-shopping" for managed care companies and others will be required to make a series of "make or buy" decisions.[5] The conventional wisdom is that hospitals will be at the top of the "food chain" when all is said and done; however, I am not quite so certain. In some locations, at least, physician groups could control the decision making and the hospital could be another cost center. Regardless, the emerging network will still have to decide whether to purchase the services of a local provider, the "buy," or, develop a program itself, the "make." These decisions will be based on several variables, many of which could be controlled, or at least influenced, by the hospice.

Certainly one of the variables will be the skill of the hospice CEO and his or her ability to identify potential partners and to participate in successful negotiations. Also to be considered is the personal interests of the hospice CEO and the CEOs of the various networks—many "win-win" scenarios are scuttled by the egos of those involved.

Obviously, public policy that dictates the inclusion of comprehensive hospice services delivered by a competent and certified provider will increase the motivation for networks to create relationships with existing hospice providers. Such relationships could result in affiliations or mergers.

An important element in this relationship building is an understanding by the network that its potential partner, the hospice program, is willing and able to share the risk of serving terminally ill patients.

By offering a comprehensive hospice benefit and negotiating a fair prospective reimbursement with the hospice, the network is able to offer an important benefit to its clients while limiting its financial risk. Given that caring for the terminally ill could pose one of the more significant financial unknowns and risks to the network, the ability to limit the unknown and share the risk with another provider should not be underestimated by the network's leadership. Bringing this issue to the attention of the network will be the responsibility of the hospice.

Third, the hospice program and its leadership will have to invest in better information generation. The old adage about "knowledge is power" is more true now than ever before. Too many in the hospice community do not know the language of health care outside of hospice care, more still do not understand the language of managed care. When providers and managed care networks know more about their business, more about the community the hospice serves, and more about the business of hospice than the hospice CEO does, the hospice program is at a negotiating disadvantage that it will unlikely overcome. This effort will require an investment in education and an investment in hardware and software to provide the best information possible about the hospice program.

Fourth, the hospice must operate in the most efficient possible manner. Such operations will require discipline and creativity. Hospice programs will be required to adopt business procedures that will reduce cost and improve productivity while at the same time improving the quality of their services.

Fifth, hospices must belong to their national and state organizations. The changing health care environment is not an event. Health care reform is rather a process, and one that will go on for a number of years at the federal and state levels. Hospices need to support national and state organizations, because hospices must be organized, present themselves in the most unified manner possible, and be prepared for the long haul. It will take the leadership of national and state hospice organizations to position hospice care for the next decade.

The critical need for creativity was mentioned earlier. National and state organizations are excellent places for training, education, and technical assistance, and such training is invaluable in focusing creative energy.

Sixth, the hospice will need to invest in its people and in their education, happiness, and loyalty. Hire the people that are going to help the hospice grow and expand its service base through their personal motivation, commitment, and creativity. Bring to these people the culture of the corporation, which should reflect the business of hospice, but more importantly the philosophy of hospice care.

Seventh, the hospice must demonstrate its commitment and ability to serve the entire community. The hospice should be considered a "community asset," but to be so considered the hospice must recruit a Board and volunteers that reflect that community. The hospice's attractiveness as a partner in new and emerging health care systems will be limited by an inability to demonstrate that it is serving the widest possible population as measured by its cultural diversity and its medical complexity. We can reduce this to the Spike Lee cliché of doing the right thing, because it is. Or we can talk about it making good business sense, because it does. But perhaps it is helpful just to think of it within the hospice philosophy of living life to its fullest. A program that creates a diverse environment provides texture, balance, and fullness to its employees, volunteers, and patients and their families.

Conversely, the hospice program that defines itself in a narrow manner and artificially limits access to its services has a low probability of survival.

Eighth, hospices must make it easy to do business with themselves. Hospices would do well to examine their business and clinical practices on a regular basis to assure that they are providing quality care in a timely and efficient manner, at a fair price.

Ninth, hospices must be absolutely ethical in their business and clinical practice. Hospices are serving the public at perhaps the most vulnerable time of their lives. The public needs to trust, without any doubt, that they are being cared for by an organization with the highest ethical standards.

Ethics start with the values of the Board and the CEO. They develop the culture that everyone else works within. Business ethics are pretty straight forward—fairness, decency, honesty, and trueness to mission. In hospice, that mission must be first and foremost the provision of the highest quality care to patients and their families. If the goal of a hospice or the individuals who lead or work there is something other than that mission, such people are well advised to seek other businesses because the hospice community does not want them, and the terminally ill do not need them.

Tenth, the success of hospice care has been due in great measure to its ability to dominate an area of service as a niche provider. Hospice providers have been successful by focusing on the terminally ill.

## ❖ Summary

The hospice cannot and should not abuse its position as a dominant provider, nor should it be inflexible in its approach to caring for people. However, there will be pressure to make hospice care all things to all people. That pressure must be resisted or hospice care may lose its identity. Hospice programs must also resist the pressure from some payers to unbundle its services, because no other provider approaches the comprehensive nature of hospice services. Hospice's ability to meet patients' needs, and its ability to save money in this health care system is keyed to the comprehensiveness of its services—anything less may actually cost money.[6]

That is not to say that a hospice provider should limit its services. To be a community asset, hospice programs should seriously consider offering services associated with end of life issues compatible with hospice care. Such services could include care to those who might be considered to be in a "preterminal" phase of a life-limiting disease; expanded bereavement programs such as school-based and bereavement camps; and public education programs associated with end of life issues.

Not all hospices will survive the next five years, fewer still the next ten years; however, for those that do survive, they will be larger, more successful, and will be rewarded in knowing that the hospice community will have achieved almost universal access to hospice care.

## ❖ References

1. Naisbitt, J. *Megatrends: Ten New Directions Transforming our Lives*. New York: Warner Books, 1982.
2. National Hospice Organization. *National Hospice Center*. National Hospice Organization, 1992.
3. Peters, T. "Crazy Times Call for Crazy Organizations." *Success*, 24A–24D; 56A–56D, July/August, 1994.
4. Harris, T.G. "The Post-capitalist Executive: An Interview with Peter F. Drucker." *Harvard Business Review*, 71(3):114–122, 1993.
5. Rubin, R.J. "Future Visions of Health Care." (Lecture presented at the National Hospice Organization Management and Leadership Conference, New Orleans, La., May 12, 1994.)
6. Manard, B., and Perrone, C. *Hospice Care: An Introduction and Review of the Evidence*. Prepared by Lewin V.H.I. for National Hospice Organization, Fairfax, VA, 1994.

## ❖ Chapter 15

# International Update

JOHN J. MAHONEY

In June, 1992, I led a delegation of physicians, nurses, social workers, and administrators to China as part of an exchange program under the auspices of the People to People organization and the Chinese Association of Science and Technology. The primary purpose of the delegation was to exchange information regarding the care of the terminally ill.

Although the information we shared with our Chinese counterparts was of the highest technical quality we probably learned a great deal more useful information from them than they did from us. We learned about the limits of the "American" model of hospice care outside of the United States. In a "home visit" to see a patient with cancer we learned about the difficulties of transportation within the city, limiting the number of patients a nurse could visit; the lack of equipment that we take for granted in the United States that makes caring for people in the home possible; and about life in a two-room apartment that would challenge even the most supportive family to care for a terminally ill person. We also learned about the impact of cultural norms on the provision of hospice care and the issues of death and dying. For example, resistance to the use of morphine for pain control in China is not simply a preference for Traditional Chinese Medicine (TCM), but is also a result of a cultural wariness of such drugs borne of the Opium Wars. Today, only certain doctors in China are permitted to prescribe narcotics in the treatment of their patients.

We also learned that the Chinese are much more grounded in the development of research to demonstrate the need for hospice care than what hospice proponents in the United States were in the early years of hospice. The National Hospice Society, located within the Tianjin Medical College, is a champion of hospice care within China, and has been a leader in developing research and educational programs promoting hospice care in China.

Every culture can teach us more about the issues of death and dying, and more and more countries can teach us about hospice care. The Hospice Information Service, a publishing unit of St. Christopher's Hospice in London, publishes a directory of hospices called *HOSPICE WORLDWIDE*. This publication lists hospices from sixty-four countries in varying stages of development.

Based on *HOSPICE WORLDWIDE*, almost weekly inquiries to our offices at NHO from newly forming hospices around the globe as well as personal interaction with national hospice associations in other countries, we can make these observations:

❖ The number of hospice programs is growing worldwide.
❖ The majority of hospice programs outside of the United States appears to be facility based, with an emphasis on inpatient care.
❖ There is an increasing interest in establishing "home care teams" as part of hospice programs, and there is a significant increase in the number of patient days that are provided in a patient's own home.
❖ Physician involvement in the development of hospice programs is much greater outside of the United States. Palliative medicine is a recognized specialty in England and specific medical school curricula have been established in England and Canada (see Chapter 16).
❖ In the United States, many hospice proponents would consider palliative medicine to be an element of hospice care. In other countries, "palliative medicine and care" is used interchangeably with the term "hospice care."
❖ Several countries have established specific hospice standards of practice.
❖ Reimbursement for hospice care is not as generous or as consistent as it is in the United States. Most countries do not have a specific reimbursement for hospice care, such as the Medicare hospice benefit.
❖ Hospices struggle to make ends meet through philanthropic support.

Hospice care in the United States is many times larger than the total of hospice care provided worldwide, whether measured in the number of hospices, the number of patients served, or the financial resources available. At some level this abundance creates a responsibility to assist in the development of hospice care around the world. In carrying out this responsibility we must remain cognizant that hospice care worldwide is not a "one size fits all" proposition. Hospice care is developing worldwide because of the increasing acceptance that hospice care is an important alternative to the types of care currently available. Even in the world's most economically distressed areas, where a case can be made that all available resources should go towards such goals as delivering potable water and creating adequate sewer systems, no one should have to die in pain, in fear, or alone.

Over the years, the National Hospice Organization (NHO) has hosted several groups from Japan, Russia, the Middle East, and Africa. We also routinely send materials overseas to developing hospices. In 1995, I lead an exchange program under the auspices of People to People, this time to Russia and Poland. NHO has also collaborated with hospice associations in Canada and Europe and is currently part of an international group studying the feasibility of a worldwide association for palliative care.

Other organizations such as the International Hospice Institute and the Academy of Hospice Physicians have also established collaborative efforts to start hospice programs in such countries as the Philippines and India. Additionally, many individuals have started personal projects to assist in the development of hospice programs abroad.

As important as being a resource to developing programs is, it is equally important that those of us who come from such abundance do not close our minds to the lessons that can be learned from our interactions with hospices in other countries. There is much for us to learn from the determination of those caring for people with AIDS in the jungle villages of Thailand, from the perseverance of the home care nurse in the teeming streets of Shanghai, and from the courage of those people starting hospice programs throughout the former Soviet Union.

In Chapter 14 of this book I wrote about the need for hospices to approach their work in a changing health care system with efficiency and creativity. Nowhere is that lesson better taught than in developing hospices around the world. The world is becoming an increasingly smaller village, and hospice care is part of that village. Those of us in the United States have much to give to emerging programs around the world and there is much that we can learn from them. If you have the opportunity to travel abroad take some time to visit the local hospice. The rewards will be far greater than your effort.

The following is a listing of national hospice associations worldwide as listed in *HOSPICE WORLDWIDE*. For further information about individual hospices in other countries you may consider contacting the national hospice association of that country or one of the following:

*Argentina*
Asociacion Argentina de Medicina
y Cuidados Paliativos
Thames 2306 1 B
Buenos Aires 1425
Argentina

*Belgium*
Federation Belge de Soins Palliatifs
217 rue Royale
Koningsstraat
1210 Bruxelles
Belgium

*China*
National Hospice Society
% Tianjin Medical College
Qixiangtal Road
Tianjin 300070
China

*Germany*
Dr. Toni Gassen Stiftung EV
Hebbelstrasse 16
Dusseldorf 1 4000
Germany

*Australia*
Australian Association for
  Hospice and Palliative Care
PO Box 1200
North Fitzroy
Victoria 3068
Australia

Federatie Terminale Zorg
Vlaanderen
Eekhoutstraat 46
Brugge 8000
Belgium

*France*
Societe Francaise
  D'Accompagnement et
  de Soins Palliatifs
110 avenue Emilie Zola
Paris 75105
France

*Great Britain*

British Soviet Hospice Association
Diary Cottage
Hitcham Lane
Burnham SL1 7DS
England

*Hong Kong*
Hong Kong Cancer Fund
10 Borrett Road
Hong Kong

*Korea*
Korea Catholic Hospice
   Association
College of Nursing—Seoul
28 YonGon-Dong
ChongNo-Ku
Seoul 110–799
Korea

*New Zealand*
Hospice New Zealand
PO Box 12481
Wellington
North Island
New Zealand

*South Africa*
Hospice Association
   of Southern Africa
PO Box 602
Durbanville 7550
Cape Province
South Africa

*Switzerland*
La Societe Suisse
   de Medecine Palliative
Fondation Rive Neuve
Clos de Moulin 20
Villeneuve CH 1884
Switzerland

The Hospice Information Service
St. Christopher's Hospice
51–59 Lawrie Park Road
Sydenham
London SE26 6DZ
England

*Italy*
The European Association
   for Palliative Care
National Cancer Institute of Milan
Via Venezian 1
Milan 20133
Italy

*Luxembourg*
Omega 90
25 Grand-Rue
L-Esch/Alzette
Luxembourg

*Poland*
National Council for Palliative
   Care/Hospice Services
c/o Palliative Care Service
Karol Marcinkowski University
   of Medical Science
ul. Lakowa 1/2
Poznan 61–878
Poland

*Spain*
Department de Sanitat
Programa Vida als Anys
Traverssera de les Corts 131–159
Barcelona 08028
Spain

*United States*
National Hospice Organization
1901 North Moore Street, Suite 901
Arlington, Virginia 22209
U.S.A.
Tel: (703) 243–5900
Fax: (703) 535–57622

## ❖ Chapter 16

# Hospice and Palliative Care in Academia

WALTER B. FORMAN

DENICE C. SHEEHAN

In the book *A Calculus of Suffering,* a chronology of the development of anesthesia, Pernick notes that with the relief of acute surgical pain using ether anesthesia the physician was freed to address the medical ethical and humanitarian issues of the day.[1] Today the medical and nursing professions, which have become highly technical pursuits, are again facing a similar opportunity. We are now technically able to save and prolong life in ways never dreamed, yet we are still faced with similar ethical and humanitarian issues that our predecessors had to confront. One of the major responses to this need has been the rapidly evolving field of palliative care. Palliative care encompasses palliative medicine, palliative nursing care, and care of the terminally ill by a variety of other professionals whose activities are reviewed in Chapters 3, 4, and 5. Palliative care has brought to the health care professions the organized structure to begin understanding the concerns and variety of symptoms suffered during a terminal illness. Like the effects of ether anesthesia on the medical profession, palliative care gives us the opportunity to return to a holistic approach to the care of the sick, as well as those with terminal illnesses. The World Health Organization has recognized the need for the development of national policies and programs for palliative care and has issued several recommendations regarding the education and training of health care professionals. In addition it has suggested that palliative care programs be incorporated into the existing health care system.[2] In this chapter the authors will define the field of palliative care, present a curriculum that will extend over the continuum of medical and nursing education, and briefly review current ongoing education in palliative care in the United States compared to other countries.

## ❖ Palliative Care: Definition and Knowledge Base

A review of Chapter 1, which summarizes the history of the hospice movement, will give the reader a fuller understanding of the emerging field of palliative health care. Early hospices were developed as a place for the terminally ill to come to die—particularly the indigent. The change in hospice that has lead to the development of the field of palliative care can be traced to one individual—Dame Cicely Saunders. In the late 1950s, she began her pioneer work to meld scientific medicine and nursing of the terminally ill. Her demonstration of the use of "round the clock" pain medication is a mile post that is the mainstay of pain management in the terminally ill cancer patient.[3] According to Derek Doyle, medical director at St. Columba's Hospice in Edinburgh, Scotland palliative medicine is the endeavor that is devoted to:

> the study and management of patients with active, progressive far advanced disease for whom the prognosis is limited and the focus of care is quality of life[4] (p. 253).

Thus, many aspects of care not usually considered traditional for physicians become important in palliative medicine. When health care professionals care for a patient for whom cure is no longer possible, they must change their goals to comfort care. They must work as a member of an interdisciplinary team, allowing the patient and family to be members of the decision-making team, dealing with the dying process and bereavement, and developing skills to become as enthusiastic about managing the dying, as they are about curing diseases. These attitudinal changes need to be accomplished in the changing environment of the health care system. The emerging modus operandi seems to favor the training of highly technical physicians and nurses. We suggest that training should be directed toward application of traditional skills along with adaptation of new technology for the care of the suffering. In addition to basic knowledge and skills, the physician must be familiar with several key areas of medical information to successfully care for the dying person. Over 80 percent of patients currently in hospice programs have cancer. Thus, the physician needs to be well versed in the areas of diagnosis and treatment of this heterogeneous disease. In addition, over 65 percent of patients are over the age of sixty-five years. Therefore, future health care professionals will need a broad knowledge of the principles of geriatric care.[5] For those involved in teaching, whether at the medical/nursing student level, postgraduate level, or in continuing medical/nursing education programs, the challenge to create relevant curriculum is now being addressed by some professional health care schools in the United States.

## ❖ Educational Programs in Palliative Care: The Problems

### The Physician

In this country, as well as in others, the development of hospice services was distinct from the traditional health care models.[6] In fact, it is more correct to state that they began as an alternative approach to the care of the dying outside of the traditional modern health care institution. The reasons for this bizarre twist that placed the care of the dying outside traditional health care is multifaceted. Death is a defeat to physicians. Thus death is ignored because it threatens the physician's knowledge, skills, and ability to cure. Second, with the advent of consumerism at the same time hospice programs appeared, the individual had an avenue to protest the tradition of dying in a hospital. To the health care field the perceived threat to its authority and financial stability was considerable. But what was the view concerning the need for information in the care of the dying? Surveys of death education in medical schools as early as the 1970s demonstrated the need to include this subject in the curriculum.[7] Plumb and Segraves surveyed postgraduate education programs in 1992. They found that of the programs that offered death education, 92 percent did so only by didactic materials—not by exposing the learner to dying patients. Mermann and colleagues did the same for medical schools in 1991.[8,9] As Mermann noted, "personal involvement of students with patients in the process of learning about death and dying was minimal, despite the widely observed fact that students can hardly wait to go on the wards" (p. 35). In 1988, Dupont noted that there was no evidence of consensus concerning course content or the need for or an attempt to integrate learning about death and dying into the training in medical, nursing, or social work schools.[10] During the last five years, surveys of practicing physicians have demonstrated their wish to increase knowledge about communicating with their dying patients. House staff have asked for more training in care of the dying.[11] In a 1992 survey of Great Britain's medical schools, Smith found in twenty-two of twenty-seven schools, medical students had a specific body of instruction in pain management and symptom control. In addition, communicating with dying patients, their families, bereavement counseling, and working in an interdisciplinary team were incorporated in the curriculum. A clinical component was present in 33 percent of the schools and in these schools all students were assigned to attend in a hospice unit. However, even with this emphasis on palliative medicine one third of the medical schools did not incorporate relevant questions on the final examination.[12] In conclusion, physicians recognized the need for instruction in palliative medicine in their daily encounters with patients and their families. Practicing physicians, medical students, and postgraduate trainees desired information in this area but it was not being taught. Fortunately, this situation in medical schools and in continuing medical education courses are dramatically changing.

## The Nurse

Care of the dying was one of the earliest responsibilities of the professional nurse. Nurses provided care to soldiers dying on the battlefields as well as to civilians dying from epidemics. A major shift in patterns of disease and treatment began in the twentieth century as more effective treatment modalities became available. Today, student nurses are exposed primarily to curative-oriented care and are less likely to encounter comfort-oriented care.[13] Quint's 1967 landmark study revealed that there was little emphasis throughout the nursing curriculum on teaching student nurses to care for dying patients.[14] As in medical schools, teaching and support was particularly lacking in the clinical setting. Nursing instructors were inadequately prepared to teach or support the students in care of the dying and were not comfortable with nursing problems associated with the dying patient. Quint recommended that faculty standardize death education curricula which could be offered consistently throughout schools of nursing, continuing education, and inservice programs.

In Webster's study, over 30 percent of the student nurses reported that they were not always told which of their patients were expected to die.[15] Additionally, 60 percent were not told whether or not the patients knew they were dying. Care of the dying patient was not routinely incorporated in their curriculum. The type and amount of knowledge and support was dependent on the instructor. Although the students may have learned these skills by working with more experienced nurses, observations revealed that 25 percent of the students worked alone with the dying. The remaining 75 percent had only intermittent supervision.[15] A review of literature by Degner and Gow in 1988 revealed that few programs in death education for nurses have been described in the literature and even fewer have been evaluated.[15]

## ❖ Educational Programs in Palliative Care: The Responses

Hospices in Great Britain and Scotland offer educational programs for physicians, nurses, clergy, and physical and occupational therapists. These programs incorporate formal didactic lectures, small group seminars, bedside instruction, apprenticeship systems for the specific professions, and multiprofessional teaching strategies. The educators at St. Columba's Hospice in Edinburgh teach awareness, general principles, and technical details.[16] Graduate diplomas in palliative care have been developed in both Great Britain and Australia. Maddocks and Donnell have instituted a program that leads to a Masters degree.[17] The program is multidisciplinary and available to graduates from any relevant field. It can be achieved at their institution in Australia or through a correspondence course. This interdisciplinary program stresses four core topics:

1. Death, society, and hospice care
2. Psychosocial aspects of palliative care
3. Practice which focuses on pain and symptom control
4. Practicum. Here the students must demonstrate at least thirty hours of field experience.

Sister Mary Cecilia Eagan and colleagues have developed an interdisciplinary hospice education program at Madonna University in Livonia, Michigan. Students may choose from four options.[18] These include:

1. A bachelor of science degree in hospice
2. An associate of science degree in hospice

3. A minor in hospice
4. A certificate of achievement in hospice

More information about these programs is provided in Appendix III.

### The Physician

The following is a review of programs that addresses the issues of palliative medicine. Curricula that deal only with death education and not the full spectrum of palliative medicine fall short of the goal. They do not emphasize the knowledge and skills necessary to control the complex symptoms of the terminally ill or address working on an interdisciplinary team. However, excellent texts such as Bertman's work *Facing Death* are recommended for teaching death education in medical schools and should be part of the palliative medicine curriculum.[19] In 1992, Knight and colleagues published a sixteen-hour curriculum for fourth year medical students which occurred during the student's family medicine clerkship.[20] Results from pretesting and posttesting showed that the curriculum had a significant effect on students' perceptions of hospice work, the benefits of hospice care, and increased their knowledge base about pain and symptom management.

The Canadian Committee on Palliative Care Education was formed in 1988 to address the issues of teaching palliative medicine in Canadian medical schools. This group, composed of two faculty members each from twelve of the sixteen medical schools in Canada, met and authored *The Canadian Palliative Care Curriculum*, published in 1991.[21] The curriculum is aimed at principles that need to be imparted to students and not at restructuring the curriculum of the medical schools. The goals of the curriculum were uniquely divided into three areas of learning: *attitude*, working in an interdisciplinary group, application of information to the therapeutic process, centering on patients' needs; *skills*, communication techniques, integration of multiple types, and sources of knowledge; and *knowledge*, understanding pathophysiology of various diseases, pharmacology as it applies to the terminally ill, and understanding grief and bereavement. These three attributes, formed here into the acronym *ASK* to emphasize the need for inquiry in palliative medicine, were used to develop an outline for symptom control, psychosocial issues, and a third topic called fundamental issues. The latter explores items such as ethics, cost, and home care. These areas are rarely addressed in medical schools.

At the same time in Great Britain, a Working Party of the Association for Palliative Medicine composed of regional educational representatives formed to develop a syllabus to teach palliative medicine. Their curriculum differs from others in that they have provided guidelines for training at three levels: medical students, generalists, and those seeking specialty certification in palliative medicine. For example, all physicians should be able to obtain a pain history. However, the generalist should know when to make a referral for pain and the palliative medicine specialist should be familiar with the above, be fluent in nondrug treatments and be able to perform common nerve blocks. The gamut of issues in palliative medicine is presented in this format and includes psychosocial issues, grief, and bereavement. To implement their curriculum at all these levels, the Working Party has added a section on where the experience should occur during training and what educational methods need to be employed.[22]

A graduate degree in palliative medicine can be obtained by correspondence and on-site experience at the University of Wales College of Medicine (see Appendix III). The call to integrate palliative medicine education into the acute hospital vis-a-vis the oncology setting is clearly delineated by Weissman, who suggests an abbreviated curriculum that addresses symptoms and ethical issues.[23] He also suggests that oncologists become the leading force in the development of palliative medicine programs. MacDonald also has presented a very excellent commentary concerning this issue.[24] In our opinion the teaching of palliative medicine is a critical component of oncology but the field of palliative medicine also must have an impact on all health care professionals. Palliative care is needed for persons with AIDS, terminal renal and hepatic failure, respiratory decompensation, and cardiac disease. Physicians in these fields must be able to provide palliative medicine for their patients.

## *The Nurse*

This section provides a review of programs that address the issues of palliative care nursing. Dicks contends that the goal of nursing care is promotion of the patient's independence or adaptation to the limitations of advancing disease.[25] In order for the nurse to assist the patient, he or she must understand the patient's needs from the patient's perspective. Therefore, good communication skills are imperative. Communication skills are an integral part of the nursing curricula. They are presented in lecture format, refined during small group discussions, and practiced in clinical settings. However, several authors have recommended that even more emphasis should be placed on communication skills.[15,26,27] Communication skills are also imperative because of the emerging role of the nurse as part of an interdisciplinary team.

Degner and Gow have described three approaches used to teach nurses to care for the dying.[26] Integrating death education into the general curriculum is the approach most often used at the undergraduate level. Graduate and continuing education programs most often present this material in an elective format. Some schools require the student to take a course on death education. Student nurses are not systematically assigned to care for dying patients, although this component is recommended in the nursing literature.

Inclusion of palliative nursing in a nursing school curriculum, as described by several authors, ranges from didactic presentations to clinical experiences.[17,26-31] Stephany, a staff nurse in hospice home care, described her experiences as a preceptor for senior baccalaureate student nurses. She spends 15 weeks with one student focusing on patient advocacy, professional accountability and holistic palliative nursing care.[30] Sorrentino described hospice care as a unique clinical experience for students in a Master of Science program in nursing. She stated that students and faculty do not usually choose hospice settings because they prefer the highly technical acute care settings. Therefore, it is important to provide students with information about hospice care that will help them to see the value of clinical experiences in this setting. The hospice clinical experience encourages a review of previously learned concepts and values. This is especially true in pain management, quality of life and the healing process.[29] Interdisciplinary approaches to death education, especially for physicians and nurses, have been recommended.[32] However, there is a paucity of articles in the literature regarding specific programs and experiences.[13] Chavasse suggests that there is a move toward a more holistic understanding of health care.[33] This understanding is being adopted as a core value in nursing curricula. This view honors the humanity of both student and patient.

A comprehensive description of a core curriculum in palliative nursing was prepared by the International Society of Nurses in Cancer Care.[27] The core curriculum has been approved by the Cancer and Palliative Care Unit of the World Health Organization as well as the International Council of Nurses. It is geared toward trained nurses rather than student nurses or advanced practice nurses in palliative care nursing. It provides a flexible framework for courses, depending on the knowledge and experience of the instructors and students, as well as the resources available.

In Canada at the University of Manitoba, Degner and Gow developed and evaluated an undergraduate course in palliative care for third-year nursing students in a baccalaureate program.[26] The course provided seventy-two hours of classes (three hours per week over two semesters) and six hours per week of supervised clinical practice. The investigators compared this group with a group of third-year nursing students who received an integrated approach to the care of the dying patient and a non-nursing control group. Student nurses, who had taken the palliative care course, had significantly better attitudes to care of the dying than those students who did not take this course. One year after graduation this group also felt more adequate in caring for dying patients. They judged their undergraduate program to be more adequate in preparing them to care for dying patients compared with the nursing control group. The investigators reported the new graduates' perceptions regarding the most effective approach to teach nursing care of the dying patient. These components include:

1. Opportunities for the students to examine their feelings in lectures and seminars.
2. An organizing framework to assist them in understanding the reactions of dying patients and their families.
3. Research-based knowledge to guide their practice.
4. Clinical assignments involving a dying patient with an opportunity to follow this patient until death and visit the family after the death.
5. Opportunities for class discussion of important clinical events.

## ❖ Curriculum Development in Palliative Medicine

1.  Where to Begin? When one considers the complexity of medical school curricula and the pressure for teaching time among the various groups vying for this time, the task of where to begin seems daunting. However, by looking at what is taught in each section of study and comparing it to the palliative medicine curriculum that you wish to introduce, an inventory of what is available and what needs to be added can evolve. Similarly, the needs of the postgraduate training programs at your institution can be approached in this manner. For this aspect of education, start with a program that is primary care oriented and one to which you have entry—for example, general medicine, family practice, or pediatrics. Review the rotations that the trainees are obligated to take for content related to the palliative care curriculum outlined below. If on the other hand you are involved in continuing medical education, a needs survey of your general audience might be a starting point.

2.  What Should Be Included in a Palliative Medicine Curriculum? As outlined by the Great Britain curriculum, it depends on the target audience. In the United States, we are far from needing a curriculum in our teaching programs that prepares an individual for specialty certification in palliative medicine. However, we do need to address the medical student and generalists' needs. Therefore, the following material should be part of a core curriculum in palliative medicine. Remember that a separate "course" does not need to be established. The material must be found somewhere in the curriculum. Although there is a sequential nature to the information, for purpose of establishing the core information we will concentrate on substance and not format. The following is "core material" for medical students, as adapted from the Working Party of the Association of Palliative Medicine

    A.  Trajectory of Chronic Progressive Diseases. It is vital that the student understands that many diseases are currently not curable or in some cases that the curative approach is merely experimental. Cancer, certain neurologic disorders, AIDS, many cardiopulmonary diseases, and hepatic/renal disorders after transplant considerations are in this category. The student should clearly know the trajectory of these disorders, therapies that alter the trajectory of the disease and to what degree, and finally, when each is no longer considered curable. For example, in reviewing the cardiovascular section of the curriculum there should be clear guidelines to the students concerning when coronary artery disease is no longer amenable to interventional therapies and medical treatments will dominate the remaining care of the patients. Here we are looking for guidance to the student from the faculty that the mode of care is changing from curing to comfort caring. What treatments will control symptoms of the disease and an indication of the pharmacology of the agents being employed, or in the case of nonpharmacologic intervention, proposed mechanism of action must be apparent. Physiology of the symptom being treated should also be evident. If pain is a part of the course of the disease a carefully thought out section should be included in this area—for example, causes of pain associated with cancer and its evaluation and management. In this example, many sections of the curriculum might have reference to this issue—oncology, neurology, pharmacology, nursing, psychology. However, there needs to be special emphasis on interdisciplinary teaching and treatment.

B.  Specific Behavioral Issues. This area can be found in many portions of the curriculum and might require some diligent searching. The students should receive instruction in:

a.  Communication Skills—breaking bad news, caring for either a dying person and/or their family, speaking with peers about difficult issues especially personal thoughts about death and dying.

b.  Ethics—a variety of issues come into play, including advanced directives, right to life status in the State, principles of ethical conduct, codes of conduct for physicians, discussion concerning euthanasia, and other similar issues.

c.  Autonomy—are students introduced to the concept of patient rights? What about individual spiritual beliefs? Do students maintain their convictions concerning spirituality outside the sick room? Do they understand cultural influences that affect decision making for both the patient and physician?

d.  The Interdisciplinary Team—the student should be exposed to working on an interdisciplinary team (nurse, social worker, cleric, and/or behavioral scientist, as a minimum).

e.  Reimbursement Issues—the student should be aware of the rules governing this topic for palliative medicine, as well as those about home care in general, medications in the home, durable medical equipment in the home, and how to submit an invoice for reimbursement.

C.  Lifelong Learning. The student should be acquainted with textbooks, journals, and other materials, such as those from the American Cancer Society and State Pain Initiatives, on an ongoing basis. In addition the student must be familiar with resources, such as the Academy of Hospice Physicians information resource, that can aid in answering questions that might arise while caring for patients. A resource list is provided in Appendix III.

D.  Experiential. At least 10 percent of the primary care rotation should be in palliative medicine. It should complement the above didactic experience. This should be a "hands-on" experience and include team meetings, home visits with a mentor, and being responsible for direct patient care.

E.   Evaluation. Examinations must be reviewed for palliative medicine content. Although it is difficult to assign a specific percentage of queries on examinations to PM, the subject should be about 10 percent of the examination in order to have an impact on learning patterns. Where oral examinations are given, a similar ratio should be employed. At the conclusion of four years of school the student should demonstrate competence in the above areas of palliative medicine.

3.   Postgraduate Training and Beyond. In 1984, Glickman evaluated the experience of thirty-one house staff in their palliative care unit.[34] The rotation stressed the above core curriculum points. Ninety-two percent of the trainees felt overall it was a valuable experience. In particular they noted increased feelings of successful management of the issues faced by terminally ill people. Of note, almost 50 percent experienced as their greatest difficulty deciding when to stop curative treatment in people with cancer. This difficult interface between acute and palliative medicine remains an issue ten years later.

The organization of a palliative care unit in an acute care teaching hospital that prides itself on cure by utilizing increasingly sophisticated techniques, presents a quandary for both the learner and the teacher. Also, with cost containment the reimbursement for palliative care beds might be less than satisfactory. With these problems in mind can we integrate this activity into the training programs of our trainees? Whether a specific unit is established or not, certainly there are people with terminal illnesses in acute care beds who could benefit from a palliative medicine consultation. We suggest that the trainees could also benefit from such a consultation. This one-on-one approach would be an initial attempt to expose trainees to palliative care.

In the United States the Veterans Administration Hospitals are required to have an interdisciplinary team available for palliative care consultations.[35] The availability of such a team in other training settings is not clear. We suggest that the next step would be to require all primary care trainees rotate with this team either during a primary care experience or preferably a month experience with the team. A syllabus should be developed to include all the elements of the program as described above for students. If possible, a palliative care unit should be developed. This is particularly important since it is the nurses, social workers, clergy, and even the housekeeping personnel that make the environment conducive for the team to function. Although attempts to form a single unit of oncology and palliative care have been undertaken, these units might neglect the issue that patients other than those with cancer need to be addressed by palliative medicine.[36,37] Special learning issues for trainees should include the ability to determine when low-tech vs. high-tech pain treatments are indicated, interdisciplinary teamwork, quality management in palliative medicine, and knowledge of reimbursement issues.

## ❖ Curriculum Development in Palliative Care Nursing

1.  Where to Begin? The amount and complexity of information being presented at the baccalaureate level seems to grow year by year. The thought of adding more content brings an audible cry from the faculty, "where and how?" Many components of palliative care nursing can be found in existing curricula. Some examples include classes on suffering and death, bioethics, and communication skills. A review of the current curriculum will reveal the content that is lacking in palliative care nursing. It is important to note that the content should be clearly defined before attempting to weave it through a curriculum. In this way, the planners may take full advantage of their vision as the conceptual framework, and add to revise courses to meet their goals. It is this author's opinion that both didactic and clinical components should begin at the sophomore level and continue through the senior level.

2.  What Should Be Included in a Palliative Nursing Curriculum? Again, the content depends on the audience. The International Society of Nurses in Cancer Care developed a core curriculum for nurses who have graduated from a basic program.[27] They suggest variations of this course for nurse specialists. The following material is suggested as part of a core curriculum in palliative nursing, as adapted from The International Society of Nurses in Cancer Care.

    A.  Nursing Care of the Client with Chronic Progressive Diseases. The student nurse should understand the symptoms related to the end stages of common diseases, such as specific cancers, congestive heart failure, neurologic disorders, and AIDS. A review of the curriculum will reveal how much of the disease process is presented. Does the content end with nursing care during the acute and chronic phases, with no mention of the final stages? For example, in reviewing the geriatric section of the curriculum, there should be a discussion regarding symptomatology during the end stages of selected disease processes. It is important to include didactic and clinical experiences which highlight the importance of a comprehensive history and physical examination as the basis for the patient's care plan. The assessment should include the physical, psychosocial, and spiritual components. For example, pain associated with lung cancer in an elderly individual may be compounded by hostility in being forced to work in a uranium mine, guilt over not quitting smoking, and loss of a spiritual connection. Pharmacologic and nonpharmacologic interventions should be discussed.

When a patient visits numerous medical specialists, the home care or hospital nurse may be the one to obtain a comprehensive list of the medications. In this example, several sections of the curriculum may have reference to this issue, including oncology, pharmacology, psychology, and geriatrics. It is important to emphasize interdisciplinary collaboration and treatment. The patient's pain may be managed by a music therapist, clergy, physician, and nurse. Each member has a different role, offering their expertise to manage the total pain. Didactic content should also include loss and grief. Physiological and psychological responses to loss should be covered as well as the characteristics of complicated grief.

B.   Specific Behavioral Issues. This content may be found in other areas of the curriculum, such as bioethics and communications. However, one should search out specific content to be sure it deals with the terminally ill patient.

   a.   Attitude—discuss and reflect on the attitudes in society to progressive illness, dying and death, including attitudes among the students.
   b.   Communication Skills—develop skills in communicating with the client, family, interdisciplinary team members, and peers.
   c.   Ethics—discuss advance directives, ethical decision making, code of conduct for nurses, euthanasia, and similar issues.
   d.   Autonomy—discuss autonomy as it relates to the nurse as patient advocate. Special emphasis should be placed on individual beliefs regarding spirituality, culture, and ethnicity.
   e.   The Interdisciplinary Team—the student should be introduced to group process in the classroom setting and work on an interdisciplinary team in the clinical setting. The clinical component should be completed with a hospice or palliative care nurse as a preceptor.
   f.   Reimbursement Issues—the student should be exposed to the guidelines for reimbursement under traditional and managed care systems for care, durable medical equipment, medications, hospitalization and respite.

C.   Lifelong Learning. The student should be acquainted with textbooks, journals, and other resources specific to palliative care. The student should also be familiar with local and national resources. A list is provided in Appendix III.

D.   Experiential. The student nurse should have at least 10 percent of clinical time in direct contact with a palliative care experience, which should complement the above didactic experience. This includes direct patient/family contact during home visits with a preceptor, team conferences, and clinical forums with the clinical group and the instructor.

E. Evaluation. Clinical evaluations should be an ongoing process that includes the student, preceptor, and instructor. Written examinations must be reviewed for palliative nursing content. Weekly clinical journals are a good way to evaluate the student's ability to assimilate the information and monitor the student's progress. It also allows the student to reflect on thoughts and feelings soon after they occur. The journals are a useful adjunct to the clinical forums.

3. Beyond the Undergraduate Program. In 1992, Sorrentino described the clinical experiences of students in a Master of Science in Nursing program.[29] This experience was an option for those students in their last clinical course that dealt with chronic care of the adult. She acknowledged the rarity of hospice clinical experiences and the importance of networking with the nurses in local hospices. Sorrentino also discussed differences between hospice and the acute care models that raised questions among the graduate students. Education is also necessary for hospice nurses. This usually begins with the orientation process that forms the framework upon which to build the necessary skills and develop the knowledge base. Ongoing opportunities include inservices, workshops, team meetings, and clinical forums within the specific hospice agency. Nurses are also encouraged to attend regional, national, and international conferences and symposiums to expand their knowledge base through formal sessions and informal networking.

## ❖ Toward Collaborative Practice among Physicians and Nurses

Many components of the medical and nursing curricula are similar. The authors suggest combined lectures, forums, and clinical experiences to share information and to begin the collaborative process prior to graduation. We need to develop faculty in the United States that can assume the responsibility for initiating these programs and instructing in their implementation. The faculty must also be able to initiate the research concerning issues of the terminally ill so that our knowledge base expands our understanding of how to care for these individuals. The most significant development in this area has been the establishment of the grants provided by the Project on Death in America through the Faculty Scholars Program. More information is provided in Appendix III. They will provide salary support for junior faculty to train and then teach palliative care. Until these individuals are ready for the challenge of producing these programs we will need to proceed with those that have an interest in the care of the terminally ill. At the least, establishing a focus group in palliative care at your institution or faculty from the various involved disciplines is a good beginning.

## ❖ Summary

This chapter has reviewed the role of hospice and palliative care in our academic institutions. It is clear that care for the terminally ill American is taking a new direction. It is hoped it will be one of changing attitudes, increasing the knowledge base concerning what happens when someone dies, and that a specific skill in caring must be part of the learning. Although this approach has concentrated on Colleges of Medicine and Nursing in the United States, Doyle in Great Britain presents another point of view. It is his contention that it is the responsibility of the local hospices to provide a clinical site and be a resource for consultation, guidance, technical advice, and understanding support. Again according to Doyle, no hospice should be established unless it is prepared to offer an education program.[16] It is Dr. Doyle's hope that in the future hospice will be revered as much for its contribution to the quality of medical and nursing practice as for its quality of patient care. The authors would add the professional hospice workers in social work, music and art therapy, and clergy to this list. The key to hospice education is competent professionals, no matter where they are working, who are willing and able to mentor students at any level in their training. We hope that our professional schools will quickly begin this task before the window of opportunity passes. With the most recent inauguration of a Faculty Scholars Program by the Project on Death in America funded by the Open Society Institute, a source of faculty to develop innovative programs in clinical care, research, education, and advocacy for the terminally ill has begun. More information on academic programs in palliative care is listed in Appendix III.

## ❖ References

1. Pernick, M.S. *A Calculus of Suffering.* New York: Columbia University Press, 1985.
2. World Health Organization. *Cancer Pain Relief and Palliative Care: Report of a WHO Expert Committee.* Geneva: World Health Organization, 1990.
3. Saunders, C. "The Evolution of the Hospices." In R.D. Mann, ed. *The History of the Management of Pain.* Park Ridge, NJ: The Parthenon Publishing Group, 1988.
4. Doyle, D. "Palliative Medicine—A Time for Definition?" *Palliative Medicine,* 7:253–255, 1993.
5. National Hospice Organization 1992 preliminary data.
6. Krant, M.J. "The Hospice Movement." *New England Journal of Medicine,* 299:546–549, 1978.
7. Schoenberg, B., and Carr, A.C. "Educating the Health Professional in the Psychosocial Care of the Terminally Ill." In A.C. Carr, B. Schoenberg and A. Katscher, eds. *Psycho-social Aspects of Terminal Care.* New York: Columbia University Press, 1972.
8. Plumb, J.D., and Segraves, M. "Terminal Care in Primary Care Postgraduate Medical Education Programs: A National Survey." *American Journal of Hospice Care,* (May/June 1992):32–35.

9. Mermann, A.C., Gunn, D.B., and Dickinson, G.E. "Learning to Care for the Dying: A Survey of Medical Schools and a Model Course." *Academic Medicine, 66:*35–38, 1991.

10. Dupont, E.M., and Francoeur, R.T. "Current State of Thanatology Education in American Health Care Professions and an Integrated Model." *Loss Grief and Care, 1 & 2:*33–38, 1988.

11. Goldberg, R., et al. "A Survey of House Staff Attitudes Toward Terminal Care Education." *Journal of Cancer Education, 2:*159–163, 1987.

12. Smith, A.M. "Palliative Medicine Education for Medical Students: A Survey of British Medical Schools, 1992." *J Med Ed, 28:*197–199, 1994.

13. Degner, L.F., and Gow, C.M. "Evaluations of Death Education in Nursing: A Critical Review." *Cancer Nursing, 11*(3):151–159, 1988.

14. Quint, J.C. *The Nurse and the Dying Patient.* New York: Macmillan, 1967.

15. Webster, N.E. "Communicating with Dying Patients." *Nursing Times,* 999–1002, June 4, 1981.

16. Doyle, D. "Hospice: An Education Center for Professionals." *Death Education, 6:*213–226, 1982.

17. Maddocks, I., and Donnell, J. "A Master's Degree and Graduate Diploma in Palliative Care." *Palliative Medicine, 6:*317–320, 1992.

18. Sr. Mary Cecilia Eagon, interview by author, June 2, 1995, Livonia, MI.

19. Bertman, S.L. *Facing Death: Images, Insights, and Interventions.* Washington, DC: Hemisphere Publishing Corp., 1991.

20. Knight, C.F., et al. "Training Our Future Physicians: A Hospice Rotation for Medical Students." *Amer J Hospice & Pall Care, 23*–28, January, February 1992.

21. The Canadian Committee on Palliative Care Education. *The Canadian Palliative Care Curriculum.* The Canadian Committee on Palliative Care Education, 1991.

22. The Working Party of the Association for Palliative Medicine. *Guidelines for Teaching of Palliative Medicine.* Great Britain: The Working Party of the Association for Palliative Medicine.

23. Weissman, D. "Palliative Medicine Education: Bridging the Gap between Acute Care and Hospice." *J Cancer Ed, 6:*67–68, 1991.

24. MacDonald, N. "Oncology and Palliative Care: The Case for Co-ordination." *Ca Treat Rev. 19,* (Supplement A):29–41, 1993.

25. Dicks, B. "The Contribution of Nursing to Palliative Care." *Palliative Medicine, 4:*197–203, 1990.

26. Degner, L.F., and Gow, C.M. "Preparing Nurses for Care of the Dying." *Cancer Nursing, 11*(3):160–169, 1988.

27. International Society of Nurses in Cancer Care. "A Core Curriculum for a Post-basic Course in Palliative Nursing." *Palliative Medicine, 4:*261–270, 1990.

28. Lev, E.L. "An Elective Course in Hospice Nursing." *Oncology Nursing Forum, 8:*27–30, 1981.

29. Sorrentino, E.A. "Hospice Care: A Unique Clinical Experience for MSN Students." *American Journal of Hospice and Palliative Care, 29*–33, January/February 1992.

30. Stephany, T.M. "Precepting a BSN Student in Home Care Hospice." *Home Healthcare Nurse, 9*(4):8, 1991.

31. Corner, J. "The Nursing Perspective." In D. Doyle, G.W.C. Hanks, and N. MacDonald, eds. *Oxford Textbook of Palliative Medicine*, Oxford: Oxford University Press, 1993.

32. Wald, F. "Terminal Care and Nursing Education," *American Journal of Nursing*, 1762–1764, October, 1979.

33. Chavasse, J. "Curriculum Evaluation in Nursing Education: A Review of the Literature." *Journal of Advanced Nursing, 19*:1024–1031, 1994.

34. Glickman, E.F., and Green, H.L. "Assessment of Resident Performance in a Hospital Based Palliative Care Unit." *Death Ed, 8*:99–111, 1984.

35. Veterans Health Administration Directive 10–92–001. "Plans for Hospice Care of the Terminally Ill Veteran." Department of Veterans Affairs. January 6, 1992.

36. MacDonald, N. "Cure and Care: Interaction between Cancer Centres and Palliative Care Units." *Recent Results in Cancer Research, 121*:399–407, 1991.

37. Barrelet, L., and Caillet-Johnson, A. M. "Organization of Palliative Care in a General Hospital." *Pall Med, 7*:39–43, 1993.

# ❖ Chapter 17
# Hospice Research

BETTY ROLLING FERRELL
BRANDI FUNK

For many, hospice and research are viewed as polar opposites. Often there exists a perspective that hospice, an intensely personal care dedicated to the terminally ill, has little need or use for the integration of research, which is viewed as an impersonal science. Others argue that the patient population involved is too ill and too vulnerable to allow meaningful scientific research and that there is not much more to find out, that the problems of pain and symptom control have been exhausted.[1] In the previous two decades of hospice development in the United States, attention has been largely focused on the concept and delivery of clinical care with less emphasis on the quantification or the science of that care. However, for many reasons, the merger of these concepts is not only beneficial to quality patient care but is also essential to the survival of hospice in the health care system.

Many observers of hospice would contend that hospice care still remains a well-guarded secret. While hospice care providers have undoubtedly made a tremendous impact on the quality of care of the dying and their families, many of these same providers have often been unable to effectively communicate the value of hospice care, attributable to the lack of research needed to quantify its true benefits. In an increasingly competitive health care system, it is essential for hospice to establish a strong financial and health policy perspective of the benefits of this care system. Thus, while the clinical future of hospice is enhanced by the demands of a chronically ill and aging population, there has never been a greater demand to integrate research into hospice care. Research must become an integral component of the development of excellent hospice care in such a way that it improves the quality of this care and justifies its future value within the broader health care system.

This chapter will discuss research as a vital component of quality hospice care. Although a full exploration of the research process is not possible within the confines of this chapter, a brief overview of various research methods and an introduction to preparing research proposals will be presented. It is the authors' intent that this chapter not be viewed as separate from the remainder of the text but rather as content that can be applied to the other clinical content. Together they will provide creative ways to improve the quality of care for the dying patient and their families and ways in which this quality of care can be quantified and effectively communicated.

## ❖ Research as a Component of Hospice Care

Research is seen as a systematic process of applying scientific methods in order to validate and refine existing knowledge and to generate new knowledge. The primary goal of nursing research is to develop a scientific knowledge base for nursing practice.[2] Though similar when applied across disciplines, the research process when applied to hospice includes some unique dimensions. Four specific goals of research in hospice can be described. The first application of research to hospice is as a means to *quantify* hospice care. Again, there remains a critical need to describe hospice care and the services provided in a way that cannot only be quantified for justification but disseminated to those yet to be converted to the hospice ideology as well.

The second purpose of hospice research is as a means of *discovery*. While some areas within hospice have been explored more thoroughly, many aspects of terminal illness and the stages of death and dying are relatively unexplored. Many of the physical and psychosocial phenomena surrounding terminal illness remain virtually void in the literature. Research should be seen as a dynamic process of discovering the critical events in the care of the terminally ill and the aspects of hospice that are most needed and beneficial to patients and families.

The third aim that can be ascribed to research in hospice is that of *quality improvement*. The field of quality assessment and improvement is in the forefront across delivery settings as systems struggle to achieve a higher quality of care within a constrained health economy. Hospice has been based on a solid foundation of which the corner stone has always been excellent patient care. A danger within the hospice community is to assume that the highest quality of care is being provided. Use of research within the quality improvement process allows hospices to continuously evaluate their own services, seek continued growth and quality improvement, and ultimately improve nursing practice.

The fourth goal of hospice research is *problem solving*. Many aspects of hospice care require a more philosophical approach in understanding existential suffering, grief, and transference from life to death. However, there are also many questions within hospice care (i.e., the best protocol for management of terminal breathlessness) that require direct answers. Application of research methods to actual patient problems enables clinicians to resolve patient care problems and to make significant contributions to the scientific basis of hospice.

## ❖ Research Designs and Methods

Many excellent resources exist to provide in-depth information regarding various research designs and methods for hospice. The diversity of care provided within hospice demands also a diversity in research approaches. Both qualitative and quantitative methods are useful to capture the outcomes of hospice. Quantitative research methods include a variety of approaches ranging from physiologic (i.e. measurement of vital signs, lab work, weight, etc.) to subjective reports by use of surveys or questionnaires. Surveys, as subjective written instruments, are perhaps the most commonly used and can serve as a valuable source of data.

Four commonly used quantitative methods include (1) descriptive, used to provide a picture of situations as they naturally occur, (2) correlational, which examines relationships between variables, (3) experimental, established for the purpose of examining causality more closely through variance control, and (4) quasi-experimental, developed to provide alternate means for examining causality in situations not conducive to experimental controls.[2,3]

Qualitative methods, such as the use of observation, patient diaries, and in-depth interviews can be very helpful to describe life experiences and give them meaning.[2] One example is the research by Raudonis which explored the meaning and impact of empathic relationships in hospice nursing using in-depth interviews which resulted in improvement and maintenance of patients' physical and emotional well-being.[4] Some common types of qualitative methods include (1) phenomenology, experiences discovered as they are lived, (2) grounded theory, theory developed from the data, (3) ethnography, an anthropologic technique of studying cultures, and (4) historical, a narrative description or analysis of events that occurred in the recent past.[2]

Retrospective data such as audit of patient records can be a practical and valuable source of hospice research.[5] For example, a retrospective review of patient records in the final forty-eight hours of life can reveal valuable information regarding symptoms experienced and interventions used and can provide the basis for further investigation and research studies. The most important consideration is to select a research design and method which is appropriate for the questions being addressed.

## ❖ Components of a Research Proposal

Extensive discussion of the research process is available in research texts, however, the following discussion will review the basic components of a research proposal (Table 17–1).[6] This content is intended as a basic guide to developing research proposals in hospice settings not currently involved in research.

### *Study Aims, Hypotheses, or Study Questions*

A research proposal begins with a statement of aims as well as study questions or hypotheses. This section conveys the goal of the study and that it should be stated as clearly and succinctly as possible. The aims or purpose should explain the needs for the study. The hypotheses or study questions focus specifically on what the researcher wants to learn. Hypotheses generally are preferred when you are predicting relationships among variables or

TABLE 17–1    Research Proposal Evaluation Criteria

*Abstract*

    Accurately reflects the proposal
    Includes problem statement and purpose
    Summarizes key variables, sample, and methods

*Study Aims, Hypotheses, or Study Questions*

    Clearly stated
    Hypotheses or study questions are consistent with the study aim

*Significance of the Study*

    Contributes to the science of hospice
    Has the potential to lead to further investigation
    The research offers a unique contribution to the literature and to hospice

*Literature Review and Theoretical Framework*

    Relevant and current literature is reviewed
    Literature primarily includes research rather than opinion
    Literature is critiqued, synthesized, and analyzed
    Framework identified is appropriate to the study and consistent with study
        questions and methods

*Subjects*

    Includes sampling method and specific procedures for identifying and selecting
        subjects
    There is evidence that adequate subjects exist
    Includes specific inclusion and exclusion criteria

*Study Design and Measurement*

    The design is appropriate for the study purpose and questions
    Addresses reliability and validity of all measurement tools
    The study design can be accomplished reasonably within the time frame
    Addresses threats to internal validity of the study

*Procedures*

    The procedures are feasible
    Includes methods for training and supervision of personnel

*Data Analysis*

    Identifies specific statistical procedures. Analysis is appropriate for the type of
        data and study design and answers the study questions.
    Describes computer facilities and consultation

*Source:* Ferrell, B.R., et al. "Applying for Oncology Nursing Society and Oncology Nursing Foundation Grants." *Oncology Nursing Forum, 16*(5):728–730, 1989.

TABLE 17-1  Research Proposal Evaluation Criteria—*Continued*

*Human Subjects Considerations*

    IRB approval is given or documentation of pending review is given

    The investigator is clearly aware of the impact of participation in the study on the subject

    Addresses concerns regarding the length, intrusiveness, and energy expenditure required

*Investigators and Research Team*

    Consultation is available for the less experienced researcher

    Establishes the role of co-investigators or consultants

---

outcomes. Study questions are more appropriate for exploratory or descriptive studies. Often, qualitative research is guided by study questions to collect data that will later generate hypotheses.

The hypotheses or study questions should flow logically from the literature review or theoretical framework and should be truly researchable. Some problems, such as ethical or moral dilemmas, simply are not answerable by scientific investigation. Questions such as, "Should withdrawal of nutrition be allowed in patients with AIDS?" are significant topics but not appropriate for research.

It is much better to create a narrow and sufficiently developed proposal rather than a broad, ambitious study that is not feasible. For example, rather than attempting to study the entire family's response to cancer deaths, the researcher might focus on a smaller dimension such as siblings' responses to death of a child with cancer.

## Significance

The significance section "sells" the proposal by convincing the reviewers that the study will contribute to patients, nurses, and/or the general healthcare community. Often, this section is weak because the investigator fails to make the significance explicit. It is important to state the significance clearly and concisely, and demonstrate how the findings will apply to future hospice care. This significance is further strengthened by explaining how it will contribute to the larger hospice community. It also is important to demonstrate how the study findings will provide a basis for future studies. This enables the reviewers to see the potentially larger contribution of this study.

## Literature Review and Theoretical Framework

The literature review presents a critical summary of what is already known about the research problem. The review should describe consistencies, contradictions, and gaps in the literature. It should be a critical analysis rather than a simple summary. With limited space, clarity and succinctness are important. Ideas should be developed logically, and the entire literature review should point to the need for the study. It is best to use the most current literature, although the review of literature can include classic or landmark studies. Use primary sources whenever possible and emphasize research literature rather than opinion.

A theoretical or conceptual framework is an important component of a proposal. Researchers often err when they present a framework but then fail to apply it to their proposed research. The investigators should describe the relationship between concepts and variables in the theory and the proposed study. A visual model is a good way to clarify these relationships for reviewers. The theory should also be reflected throughout the proposal. For example, a theoretical framework should lend direction to the study questions and should be consistent with the methods and instruments used.

## Subjects

This section of a proposal addresses the type and number of subjects to be used as well as their availability and accessibility to the investigator. This includes a description of the study setting, subject criteria, procedures for subject selection, estimate of available subjects, and the sample size. In hospice care, it is essential that attrition is considered due to deaths. This is usually anticipated by oversampling for the actual number of subjects needed. It is helpful to support availability with relevant data from past experience, such as numbers of new patients in the prior year or comparisons to other similar studies that have been accomplished in the setting.

When the design includes comparisons between groups or points in time, a power analysis allows evaluation of the magnitude of differences needed based on projected sample size. [7,8] Small samples may not detect a difference that exists, while unnecessarily large samples may produce little increase in power and, therefore, may not be cost effective.

## Measurement

This section is an important part of the study methods in establishing how all dependent variables, items when changed do so in relation to another item, will be measured. It is often helpful to indicate if the study instruments have been used in hospice studies or similar frail populations. Multiple measures of a variable (i.e., two different forms of assessing grief response) may be a strength if they do not impose undue burdens on subjects.

Because minimal research has been done is some areas of hospice, it is often necessary to develop or test new instruments. When the purpose of the study is to develop, test, and/or revise an instrument or measure, the measurement section of the proposal requires extensive discussion of psychometric issues. Psychometric testing should include multiple methods of establishing reliability and validity.

## Procedures

Proposals are enhanced when the procedures are described in a step-by-step approach. Present the processes used to identify and recruit subjects, manipulate the independent variable, and collect data. Include a timetable for the total project. Identify study limitations, factors which the study cannot address. It is very important for investigators to acknowledge their limitations in advance. A common limitation in hospice research is small sample size. A table can be used to identify complex interventions or to describe data collection procedures. In a qualitative study, this section contains information about observational or interview procedures used to obtain data and the method of recording or retrieving these data for analysis.

This section is critical in the reviewers' evaluation of the internal validity of the study. The procedures should convince the reviewers that the investigator has established control features in the study methods. Copies of protocols, such as interventions, can be included as an appendix. A small pilot study of the proposed procedures can be a strength in demonstrating that the procedures are feasible. While methods used in qualitative and quantitative studies differ, reviewers use the description of procedures in either case to determine the extent of the investigator's understanding of the complex issues surrounding the implementation of the study and the potential for successful completion.[9]

## Data Management

The proposal should clearly describe methods for data entry and analysis. Use of a statistical consultant is preferred unless the investigator has documented expertise in this area. The description of data analysis should include exact statistical procedures that are appropriate, and the analysis plan should account for all data collected. Data analysis should answer the research hypotheses or questions. Often investigators plan on including a statistician if the proposal is funded. Involving a statistician in preparing the proposal greatly strengthens the likelihood of success.

## Investigators and the Research Team

The researcher should be aware of personal strengths and limitations to include appropriate support from co-investigators or consultants to the project. Much like a hospice clinical team, the research team should demonstrate combined strength. The previous experience of these team members is important and should be related to the proposed study. Consultants and co-investigators should demonstrate their interest in your project through letters of support, and be very precise about what they will contribute. Co-investigators generally are more involved throughout the project and are listed and reimbursed by their percent of effort over the course of the study.

Consultants have more limited involvement, often on an as-needed basis, described by the number of hours or days to be used, and are paid on an hourly rate. Use of a known expert in the field as a consultant can be an asset to the proposal but the investigator must clearly describe what that expert will do, rather than simply present the expert's name to enhance the proposal. Consultants or co-investigators should review the proposal before its submission. Table 17–2 provides general tips for grant writing.[6]

## ❖ Challenges in Conducting Hospice Research

Hospice is an area of great opportunity for research and yet also one of the most challenging of environments in which to conduct research. There are many barriers to hospice research, yet investigators have demonstrated that these are surmountable and that the challenge is worth the reward of communicating the benefits of hospice. The first and foremost challenge is to recognize that hospice is a form of care, and as such, research will always be second priority. Research cannot compromise the quality of care that is embodied by hospice. The experiences of the terminal phase of life are some of the most intense of life's emotions. Family caregiving for loved ones in pain, facing death, and the loss of one's own life or grief for another are intense human experiences that are difficult to capture by the best of researchers or methods.

Extreme sensitivity is required in hospice research and is best accomplished by collaboration between clinicians and researchers. For example, in

TABLE 17–2  General Tips for Grantwriting

1. Grantwriting is not a solo activity—seek consultation and collaboration from others.

2. Have your proposal reviewed by peers before submitting it for funding.

3. Follow the directions in detail including margins, page limits, and the use of references or appendices.

4. State ideas clearly and succinctly. Give attention to spelling and grammar.

5. Use letter quality printing rather than dot matrix and use a good quality copier.

6. Plan ahead and develop a time frame for completing your grant. Avoid the last minute rush that will compromise the quality of your proposal.

7. Use appendices to include study instruments, procedures, or other supporting materials.

8. Include support letters from individuals who are important to the success of your study. This includes medical staff, nursing administration, consultants, and co-investigators.

*Source:* Ferrell, B.R., et al. "Applying for Oncology Nursing Society and Oncology Nursing Foundation Grants." *Oncology Nursing Forum,* 16(5):728–730, 1989.

our own research we have insisted on using only registered nurses with hospice or similar clinical experiences to be involved in any data collection activities. Use of qualitative methods to allow for expression of the true experience of terminal illness by those experiencing it has also enhanced work in this area.

An additional area of challenge for hospice research is the reality of constrained resources. Most hospices are challenged to provide the direct clinical care with limited resources available. Limited funds are available to support even small research projects. Thus, for any hospice, successful integration of research will be based on a realistic approach in establishing a track record of successful pilot studies before attempting larger, more complex or longitudinal designs. Hospice research is best accomplished using an interdisciplinary approach and by addressing areas that will have a direct impact on patient and family care.

## ❖ Areas of Future Research in Hospice

Finding a research problem, the first step in the scientific process, should not only reflect a situation in need of a solution, improvement, or alteration but an area of personal interest to the researcher.[2] Review of hospice research to date reveals important contributions in areas such as pain but many areas where much study is still needed. Those studies most unique to hospice include volunteerism, spiritual care, grief, emotional factors hindering symptom control, and long-term effectiveness of bereavement care.[10] The reader is referred to Appendix IIIC for a list of journals which publish peer-reviewed hospice and palliative care research.

## ❖ Summary

Most hospices have built a record of excellence of patient care using a calculated approach of small steps and by combining the strength of volunteers and professionals. Success in research is very similar. However, the main challenge to hospice and palliative care is to incorporate research into clinical practice. For example, do combinations of antiemetic medications in suppository form compounded by the local pharmacist provide effective control of nausea and vomiting as well as meet the rigid criteria necessary for all new drug formulations? What are the criteria for valid advanced directives in the hospice setting?

## ❖ References

1. Doyle, D., Hanks, G.W.C., and MacDonald, N., eds. *Oxford Text of Palliative Medicine.* Oxford: Oxford University Press, 1993.
2. Burns, N., and Grove, S. *The Practice of Nursing Research: Conduct, Critique, and Utilization,* 3rd ed. Philadelphia: W.B. Saunders, 1993.

3. Polit, D.F., and Hungler, B.P. *Essentials of Nursing Research: Methods, Appraisal and Utilization,* 3rd ed. Philadelphia: J.B. Lippincott, 1993.
4. Raudonis, B.M. "The Meaning and Impact of Empathic Relationships in Hospice Nursing." *Cancer Nursing, 16*(4):304–309, 1993.
5. LoBiondo-Wood, G., and Haber, J. *Nursing Research: Methods, Critical Appraisal, and Utilization,* 3rd ed. St. Louis: Mosby, 1994.
6. Ferrell, B.R., et al. "Applying for Oncology Nursing Society and Oncology Nursing Foundation Grants." *Oncology Nursing Forum, 16*(5):728–730, 1989.
7. Kreamer, H., and Thiemann, S. *How Many Subjects? Statistical Power Analysis in Research.* Newbury Park, CA: Sage, 1987.
8. Cohen, J. *Statistical Power Analysis for the Behavioral Sciences.* New York: Academic Press, 1977.
9. Sandelowski, M., Davis, D., and Harris, B. "Artful Design: Writing the Proposal for Research in the Naturalist Paradigm." *Research in Nursing Health,* 12(2):77–84, 1989.
10. Groenwald, S. L., et al. *Cancer Nursing: Principles and Practice,* 3rd ed. Boston: Jones and Bartlett, 1993.

# ❖ Appendix I
## Assessment Tools

- ❖ Initial Pain Assessment Tool
- ❖ Brief Pain Inventory (Short Form)
- ❖ Memorial Pain Assessment Card
- ❖ Pain Distress Scales
- ❖ Katz Index of Independence in Activities of Daily Living
- ❖ The Five Instrumental Activities of Daily Living Items, Adapted from the OARS Multidimensional Functional Assessment Questionnaire

# Initial Pain Assessment Tool

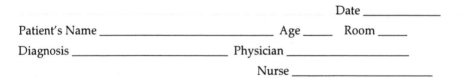

Date _____

Patient's Name _____ Age _____ Room _____

Diagnosis _____ Physician _____

Nurse _____

I. LOCATION: Patient or nurse mark drawing

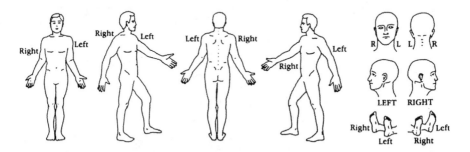

II. INTENSITY: Patient rates the pain. Scale used _____

    Present: _____
    Worst pain gets: _____
    Best pain gets: _____
    Acceptable level of pain: _____

III. QUALITY: (Use patient's own words, e.g. prick, ache, burn, throb, pull, sharp)
    _____
    _____

IV. ONSET, DURATION, VARIATIONS, RHYTHMS: _____
    _____

V. MANNER OF EXPRESSING PAIN: _____
    _____
    _____

VI. WHAT RELIEVES THE PAIN? _____
    _____
    _____

VII. WHAT CAUSES OR INCREASES THE PAIN? _____
    _____
    _____

VIII. EFFECTS OF PAIN: (Note decreased function, decreased quality of life.)

    Accompanying symptoms (e.g. nausea) _____
    Sleep _____
    Appetite _____
    Physical activity _____

Relationships with others (e.g. irritability) _____

Emotions (e.g. anger, suicidal, crying) _____

Concentration _____

Other _____

IX    OTHER COMMENTS: _____

_____

X.    PLAN: _____

_____

*Source:* From McCaffery, M., and Bebe, A. *Pain: Clinical Manual for Nursing Practice.* St. Louis: The C.V. Mosby Company, 1989. May be duplicated for use in clinical practice.

# Brief Pain Inventory (Short Form)

Study ID # _____          Hospital # _____

Do not write above this line

Date: _____/_____/_____

Time: _____

Name: _____     _____     _____
               Last                              First                         Middle Initial

1) Throughout our lives, most of us have had pain from time to time (such as minor headaches, sprains, and toothaches). Have you had pain other than these every-day kinds of pain today?     1. Yes     2. No

2) On the diagram, shade in the areas where you feel pain. Put an X on the area that hurts the most.

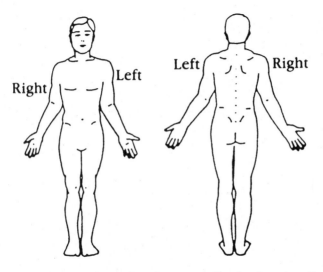

3) Please rate your pain by circling the one number that best describes your pain at its **worst** in the past 24 hours.

| 0 | 1 | 2 | 3 | 4 | 5 | 6 | 7 | 8 | 9 | 10 |
|---|---|---|---|---|---|---|---|---|---|----|
No                                                         Pain as bad as
pain                                                       you can imagine

4) Please rate your pain by circling the one number that best describes your pain at its **least** in the past 24 hours.

| 0 | 1 | 2 | 3 | 4 | 5 | 6 | 7 | 8 | 9 | 10 |
|---|---|---|---|---|---|---|---|---|---|----|
No                                                         Pain as bad as
pain                                                       you can imagine

5) Please rate your pain by circling the one number that best describes your pain on the **average.**

| 0 | 1 | 2 | 3 | 4 | 5 | 6 | 7 | 8 | 9 | 10 |
|---|---|---|---|---|---|---|---|---|---|----|
No                                                         Pain as bad as
pain                                                       you can imagine

6) Please rate your pain by circling the one number that tells how much pain you have **right now**.

| 0 | 1 | 2 | 3 | 4 | 5 | 6 | 7 | 8 | 9 | 10 |
|---|---|---|---|---|---|---|---|---|---|----|

No
pain

Pain as bad as
you can imagine

7) What treatments or medications are you receiving for your pain?

_____

8) In the past 24 hours, how much **relief** have pain treatments or medications provided? Please circle the one percentage that most shows how much relief you have received.

| 0% | 10% | 20% | 30% | 40% | 50% | 60% | 70% | 80% | 90% | 100% |
|----|-----|-----|-----|-----|-----|-----|-----|-----|-----|------|

No
relief

Complete
relief

9) Circle the one number that describes how, during the past 24 hours, **pain has interfered** with your:

A. General activity

| 0 | 1 | 2 | 3 | 4 | 5 | 6 | 7 | 8 | 9 | 10 |
|---|---|---|---|---|---|---|---|---|---|----|

Does not
interfere

Completely
interferes

B. Mood

| 0 | 1 | 2 | 3 | 4 | 5 | 6 | 7 | 8 | 9 | 10 |
|---|---|---|---|---|---|---|---|---|---|----|

Does not
interfere

Completely
interferes

C. Walking ability

| 0 | 1 | 2 | 3 | 4 | 5 | 6 | 7 | 8 | 9 | 10 |
|---|---|---|---|---|---|---|---|---|---|----|

Does not
interfere

Completely
interferes

D. Normal work (includes both work outside the home and housework)

| 0 | 1 | 2 | 3 | 4 | 5 | 6 | 7 | 8 | 9 | 10 |
|---|---|---|---|---|---|---|---|---|---|----|

Does not
interfere

Completely
interferes

E. Relations with other people

| 0 | 1 | 2 | 3 | 4 | 5 | 6 | 7 | 8 | 9 | 10 |
|---|---|---|---|---|---|---|---|---|---|----|

Does not
interfere

Completely
interferes

F. Sleep

| 0 | 1 | 2 | 3 | 4 | 5 | 6 | 7 | 8 | 9 | 10 |
|---|---|---|---|---|---|---|---|---|---|----|

Does not
interfere

Completely
interferes

G. Enjoyment of life

| 0 | 1 | 2 | 3 | 4 | 5 | 6 | 7 | 8 | 9 | 10 |
|---|---|---|---|---|---|---|---|---|---|----|

Does not
interfere

Completely
interferes

*Source:* Pain Research Group. Department of Neurology, University of Wisconsin-Madison. Used with permission. May be duplicated and used in clinical practice.

## Memorial Pain Assessment Card

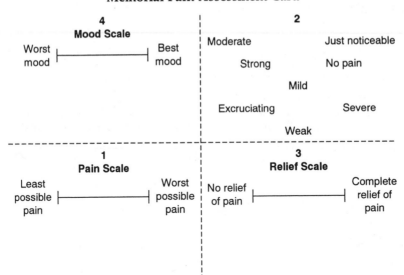

*Note:* Card is folded along broken line so that each measure is presented to the patient separately in the numbered order.
*Source:* Fishman, B., Pasternak, S., Wallenstein, S.L., et al. The Memorial Pain Assessment Card: A Valid Instrument for the Evaluation of Cancer Pain. *Cancer,* 60(5):1151–1158. 1987. Used with permission.

## Pain Distress Scales

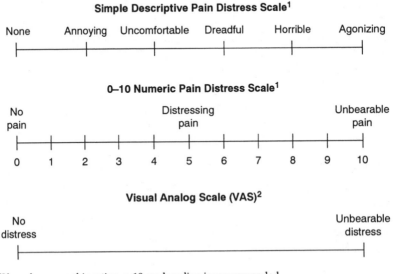

[1]If used as a graphic rating, a 10-cm baseline is recommended.
[2]A 10-cm baseline is recommended for VAS scales.
*Source:* Acute Pain Management Guideline Panel, 1992.

# Katz Index of Independence in Activities of Daily Living

The Index of Independence in Activities of Daily Living is based on an evaluation of the functional independence or dependence of patients in bathing, dressing, going to toilet, transferring, continence, and feeding. Specific definitions of functional independence and dependence appear below the index.

- A — Independent in feeding, continence, transferring, going to toilet, dressing, and bathing.
- B — Independent in all but one of these functions.
- C — Independent in all but bathing and one additional function.
- D — Independent in all but bathing, dressing, and one additional function.
- E — Independent in all but bathing, dressing, going to toilet, and one additional function.
- F — Independent in all but bathing, dressing, going to toilet, transferring, and one additional function.
- G — Dependent in all six functions.

Other — Dependent in at least two functions, but not classifiable as C, D, E, or F.

Independence means without supervision, direction, or active personal assistance, except as specifically noted below. This is based on actual status and not on ability. A patient who refuses to perform a function is considered as not performing the function, even though he is deemed able.

**Bathing (Sponge, Shower, or Tub)**
Independent: assistance only in bathing a single part (as back or disabled extremity) or bathes self completely
Dependent: assistance in bathing more than one part of body; assistance in getting in or out of tub or does not bathe self

**Dressing**
Independent: gets clothes from closets and drawers; puts on clothes, outer garments, braces; manages fasteners; act of tying shoes is excluded
Dependent: does not dress self or remains partly undressed

**Going to Toilet**
Independent: gets to toilet; gets on and off toilet; arranges clothes; cleans organs of excretion; (may manage own bedpan used at night only and may or may not be using mechanical supports)
Dependent: uses bedpan or commode or receives assistance in getting to and using toilet

**Transfer**
Independent: moves in and out of bed independently and moves in and out of chair independently (may or may not be using mechanical supports)
Dependent: assistance in moving in or out of bed and/or chair: does not perform one or more transfers

**Continence**
Independent: urination and defecation entirely self-controlled
Dependent: partial or total incontinence in urination or defecation; partial or total control by enemas, catheters, or regulated use of urinals and/or bedpans

**Feeding**
Independent: gets food from plate or its equivalent into mouth; (precutting of meat and preparation of food, as buttering bread, are excluded from evaluation)
Dependent: assistance in act of feeding (see above); does not eat at all or parenteral feeding

Source: Katz, S., Ford, A.B., et al. The Index of ADL: A Standardized Measure of Biological and Psychosocial Function. *JAMA, 185*:914–919, Sept. 21, 1963. Copyright 1963, American Medical Association.

## Evaluation Form

Name _____    Date of evaluation _____

For each area of functioning listed below, check description that applies. (The word "assistance" means supervision, direction or personal assistance.)

Bathing—either sponge bath, tub bath, or shower

☐

Receives no assistance (gets in and out of tub by self if tub is usual means of bathing)

☐

Receives assistance in bathing only one part of the body (such as back or a leg)

☐

Receives assistance in bathing more than one part of the body (or not bathed)

Dressing—gets clothes from closets and drawers—including under clothes, outer garments and using fasteners (including braces worn)

☐

Gets clothes and gets completely dressed without assistance

☐

Gets clothes and gets dressed without assistance except for assistance in tying shoes

☐

Receives assistance in getting clothes or in getting dressed, or stays partly or completely undressed

Toileting—going to the "toilet room" for bowel and urine elimination; cleaning self after elimination, and arranging clothes

☐

Goes to "toilet room," cleans self, and arranges clothes without assistance (may use object for support such as cane, walker, or wheelchair and may manage night bedpan or commode, emptying same in morning)

☐

Receives assistance in going to "toilet room" or in cleansing self or in arranging clothes after elimination or in use of night bedpan or commode

☐

Doesn't go to room termed "toilet" for the elimination process

Transfer—

☐

Moves in and out of bed as well as in and out of chair without assistance (may be using object for support such as cane or walker)

☐

Moves in or out of bed or chair with assistance

☐

Doesn't get out of bed

Continence—

☐

Controls urination and
bowel movement com-
pletely by self

☐

Has occasional
"accidents"

☐

Supervision helps keep
urine or bowel control;
catheter is used, or is
incontinent

Feeding—

☐

Feeds self without
assistance

☐

Feeds self except for getting assistance in cutting
meat or buttering bread

☐

Receives assistance in
feeding or is fed partly or
completely by using tubes
or intravenous fluids

### The Five Instrumental Activities of Daily Living Items, Adapted from the OARS Multidimensional Functional Assessment Questionnaire

1. Can you get to places out of walking distance . . .
   1 Without help (can travel alone on buses, taxis, or drive your own car),
   0 With some help (need someone to help you or go with you when traveling), or are you unable to travel unless emergency arrangements are made for a specialized vehicle like an ambulance?
   – Not answered

2. Can you go shopping for groceries or clothes (assuming she or he has transportation) . . .
   1 Without help (taking care of all shopping needs yourself, assuming you had transportation),
   0 With some help (need someone to go with you on all shopping trips), or are you completely unable to do any shopping?
   – Not answered

3. Can you prepare your own meals . . .
   1 Without help (plan and cook full meals yourself),
   0 With some help (can prepare some things but unable to cook full meals yourself), or are you completely unable to prepare any meals?
   – Not answered

4. Can you do your housework . . .
   1 Without help (can scrub floors, etc.),
   0 With some help (can do light housework but need help with heavy work), or are you completely unable to do any housework?
   – Not answered

5. Can you handle your own money . . .
   1 Without help (write checks, pay bills, etc.),
   0 With some help (manage day-to-day buying but need help with managing your checkbook and paying your bills), or are you completely unable to handle money?
   – Not answered

Source: Fillenbaum, G.G. Screening the Elderly: A Brief Instrumental Activities of Daily Living Measure. Journal of the American Geriatrics Society, 33(10):698–706, 1985.

# ❖ Appendix II
# Pain Diary

❖ Daily Diary
❖ Pain Management Log

## Daily Diary

Name _____     Date _____

| Time | Pain rating scale | Medication type & amount taken | Other pain relief measures tried or anything that influences your pain | Major activity being done: lying, sitting, standing/walking |
|---|---|---|---|---|
| 12 MIDNIGHT | | | | |
| 1 AM | | | | |
| 2 | | | | |
| 3 | | | | |
| 4 | | | | |
| 5 | | | | |
| 6 | | | | |
| 7 | | | | |
| 8 | | | | |
| 9 | | | | |
| 10 | | | | |
| 11 | | | | |
| 12 NOON | | | | |
| 1 | | | | |
| 2 | | | | |
| 3 | | | | |
| 4 | | | | |
| 5 | | | | |
| 6 | | | | |
| 7 | | | | |
| 8 | | | | |
| 9 | | | | |
| 10 | | | | |
| 11 | | | | |

Comments: _____

*Source:* From McCaffery, M., and Bebe, A. *Pain: Clinical Manual for Nursing Practice.* St. Louis: The CV Mosby Company, 1989. May be duplicated for use in clinical practice.

## Pain Management Log

Pain management log for

Please use this pain assessment scale to fill out your pain control log:

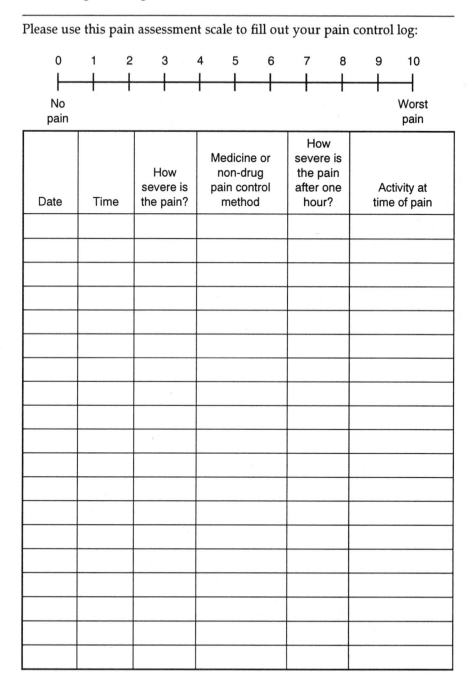

| Date | Time | How severe is the pain? | Medicine or non-drug pain control method | How severe is the pain after one hour? | Activity at time of pain |
|------|------|------|------|------|------|
|  |  |  |  |  |  |
|  |  |  |  |  |  |
|  |  |  |  |  |  |
|  |  |  |  |  |  |
|  |  |  |  |  |  |
|  |  |  |  |  |  |
|  |  |  |  |  |  |
|  |  |  |  |  |  |
|  |  |  |  |  |  |
|  |  |  |  |  |  |
|  |  |  |  |  |  |
|  |  |  |  |  |  |
|  |  |  |  |  |  |
|  |  |  |  |  |  |
|  |  |  |  |  |  |
|  |  |  |  |  |  |
|  |  |  |  |  |  |
|  |  |  |  |  |  |
|  |  |  |  |  |  |

# ❖ Appendix III
# Resources

## ❖ Organizations

Academy of Hospice Nurses
32478 Dunford Road
Farmington Hills, MI 48334

American Association
  of Music Therapy
P.O. Box 80012
Valley Forge, PA 19484

American Society of Pain
  Management Nurses
P.O. Box 2162
Tucker, GA 30085

Association of Oncology
  Social Work
1910 E. Jefferson Street
Baltimore, MD 21205

Hospice Nurses Association
5512 Northumberland Street
Pittsburgh, PA 15217-1131

National Association
  of Music Therapy
8455 Colesville Road
Suite 930
Silver Springs, MA
  20910-3392

Academy of Hospice
  Physicians
P.O. Box 14288
Gainesville, FL 32604-2288

American Pain Society
5700 Old Orchard Road
Skokie, IL 60077-1057

Association for Death
  Education and Counseling
638 Prospect Avenue
Hartford, CT 06105-4298

Choice in Dying
200 Varick Street, 10th Floor
New York, NY 10014-4810

International Hospice Institute
1275 K Street NW
10th Floor
Washington, DC 20005

National Hospice Organization
1901 North Moore, Suite 901
Arlington, VA 22209
Hospice Helpline 1-800-658-8898

Oncology Nursing Society
501 Holiday Drive
Pittsburgh, PA 15220-2749

World Health Organization
Geneva, Switzerland
To order publications:
WHO Publications Center USA
49 Sheridan Ave.
Albany, NY 12210

Resource Center for State
  Cancer Pain Initiatives
3671 Medical Sciences Center
1300 University Avenue
Madison, WI 53706
http//www.biostat.wisc.edu/
  WIIcancerpain

## *Educational Resources*

Hospice Link
Hospice Education Institute
190 Westbrook Road
Essex, CT 06426-1511
1-800-331-1620

U.S. Department of Health
  and Human Services
Agency for Health Care Policy
  and Research (AHCPR)
Willco Building Suite 310
6000 Executive Boulevard
Rockville, MD 20852
1-800-358-9295

Roxane Pain Institute
Roxane Laboratories, Inc.
P.O. Box 16532
Columbus, OH 43216
1-800-335-9100
http://www.Roxane.com

## ❖ Books

Callahan, D. *The Troubled Dream of Life: Living with Mortality.* New York: Simon and Schuster, 1993.

Chapman, C.R., and Bonica, J.J., eds. *Cancer Pain.* Kalamazoo: Upjohn Co., 1992.

Corless, I.B., Germino, B.B. and Pittman, M., eds. *A Challenge for Living: Death, Dying and Bereavement.* Boston: Jones and Bartlett, 1995.

Corless, I.B., Germino, B.B., and Pittman, M., eds. *Dying, Death, and Bereavement: Theoretical Perspectives and Other Ways of Knowing.* Boston: Jones and Bartlett, 1994.

Doyle, D., Hanks, G.W.C., and MacDonald, N., eds. *Oxford Textbook of Palliative Medicine.* Oxford: Oxford University Press, 1993.

Enck, R.E. *The Medical Care of Terminally Ill Patients.* Baltimore: Johns Hopkins University Press, 1994.

Johanson, G. *Physician's Handbook of Symptom Relief in Terminal Care,* 4th ed. Santa Rosa: Sonoma County Academic Foundation for Excellence in Medicine, 1993.

Kaye, P. *Notes on Symptom Control in Hospice and Palliative Care.* Essex: Hospice Education Institute, 1989.

McCaffery, M., and Bebe, A. *Pain: Clinical Manual for Nursing Practice*. St. Louis: C.V. Mosby, 1989.

McGuire, D., Yarbro, C.H., and Ferrell, B.R. *Cancer Pain Management*, 2nd ed. Boston: Jones and Bartlett, 1995.

Twycross, R., ed. *Pain Relief in Advanced Cancer*. London: Churchill-Livingstone, 1994.

Twycross, R.G., and Lack, S.A., eds. *Therapeutics in Terminal Cancer*, 2nd ed. London: Churchill-Livingstone, 1990.

Walsh, T.D. *Symptom Control*. Cambridge: Blackwell, 1989.

Watt-Watson, J.H., and Donovan, M.I., eds. *Pain Management: Nursing Perspective*. St. Louis: Mosby–Year Book, 1992.

Woodruff, R. *Palliative Medicine*. Melbourne: Asperula Pty. Ltd., 1993.

## Booklets

American Pain Society. *Principles of Analgesic Use in the Treatment of Acute Pain and Cancer Pain*, 3rd ed. Skokie, IL: American Pain Society, 1992.

Jacox, A.K., Carr, D.B., and Payne, R., et al. *Management of Cancer Pain. Clinical Practice Guideline Number 9*. Rockville, MD: Agency for Health Care Policy and Research, 1994.

Storey, P. *Primer of Palliative Care*. Gainesville: Academy of Hospice Physicians, 1994.

World Health Organization. *Cancer Pain Relief*. Geneva: World Health Organization, 1986.

## ❖ Journals

*American Journal of Hospice and Palliative Care*
Prime National Publishing Corp.
470 Boston Post Road
Weston, MA 02193

*Hospice Journal*
National Hospice Organization
1901 North Moore, Suite 901
Arlington, VA 22209

*Journal of Palliative Care*
Clinical Research Institute of Montreal
Center for Bioethics
110 Pine Ave.
Montreal, Quebec H2W 1R7
Canada

*Cancer Pain Release* (newsletter)
1900 University Avenue
Madison, WI 53705

*International Journal of Palliative Nursing*
Subscriptions Dept.
Mark Allen Publishing, Ltd.
Crowted Mews
286A–288 Croxted Road
London, SE24 9BY
United Kingdom

*Journal of Pain and Symptom Management*
Elsevier Science, Inc.
P.O. Box 882
New York, NY 10159

*Palliative Care Letter*
Roxane Laboratories, Inc.
P.O. Box 16532
Columbus, OH 43216

*Progress in Palliative Care*
Publications Subscription Dept.
Royal Society of Medicine
   Press Limited
P.O. Box 9002
London W1A OZA
United Kingdom

*Palliative Medicine*
Edward Arnold Ltd.
41 Bedford Square
London WC1B 3DQ
United Kingdom

*The Western Journal of Medicine,*
   Vol. 163, No. 3, 1995
Cassell, C.K., and
   Omenn, G.S., eds.
Entire volume on caring for
   patients at the end of life.
Circulation: P.O. Box 7602
San Francisco, CA 94120-7602

## ❖ Palliative Care Academic Programs

### *Memorial Sloan-Kettering Cancer Center*

Special elective for nurses, residents, and fellows in cancer pain management and supportive care:

Mary Callaway
Education Coordinator, Pain Service
Memorial Hospital
1275 York Avenue
Box 52
New York, NY 10021

The Network Project:

❖ Cancer education and training program in pain management, rehabilitation, and psychosocial issues
❖ 1–2 week observership for physicians, nurses, social workers, and occupational and physical therapists

William Breitbart, MD
Memorial Sloan-Kettering Hospital
Box 421
1275 York Avenue
New York, NY 10021

### *The Cleveland Clinic Foundation*

The Scholar's Program in Palliative Care:

❖ Internships for physicians, nurses, and pharmacists

The Cleveland Clinic Palliative Care Program:

❖ One year clinical/research fellowships

Dr. T. Declan Walsh, MSc
Director, Palliative Care Services T-33
The Cleveland Clinic Foundation
9500 Euclid Avenue
Cleveland, OH 44195

## The Hospice at the Texas Medical Center and the MD Anderson Cancer Center

❖ One year fellowships for physicians:

Porter Storey, MD
The Hospice at the Texas Medical Center
1905 Holcombe Blvd.
Houston, TX 77030

## Interdisciplinary Hospice Program

Sister Mary Cecilia Eagan, PhD, MSN
Madonna University
36600 Schoolcraft Road
Livonia, MI 48150-1171

## A Master's Degree and Graduate Diploma in Palliative Care

Ian Maddocks
Professor of Palliative Care
Daw House Hospice
Daw Park, South Australia 5041
Australia

## Diploma in Palliative Medicine

University of Wales College of Medicine
The Course Secretary, Marie Curie Centre
HOLME Tower Bridgeman Road
Penarth, South Glamorgan, CF64 3YR

## A Fellowship Program in Palliative Medicine

Department of Oncology, University of Alberta
Dr. Eduardo Bruera

Division of Palliative Care Medicine
Edmonton General Hospital
11111 Jasper Avenue
Edmonton, AB T5K 0L4
Canada

## ❖ Grants

The Project on Death in America
Dr. Susan Block
Open Society Institute
888 Seventh Avenue
19th Floor
New York, NY 10106

National Hospice Foundation
1901 North Moore, Suite 901
Arlington, VA 22209

National Cancer Institute
9030 Old Georgetown Road
Bethesda, MD 20814-1519

Oncology Nursing Society
501 Holiday Drive
Pittsburgh, PA 15220-2749

## ❖ Other

Internet search: Palliative Care

# Index

Acute care criteria, 54
Adjuvant analgesics, 76, 77, 78
  for cancer associated pain, 79
Advance directives
  general background of, 120–122
  in palliative care, 122–123
Aide, health, home, 41–43
AIDS residences, 59
Analgesics, adjuvant, 76, 77, 78
  for cancer associated pain, 79
Anorexia/nausea/emesis, 86–88
Art therapist, 46–47
Ascites, 90
Assessment nurse, 35
Attending physician, 34
Attributes of a hospice nurse, 35
Average hospice patient census
  1990, 13

Benchmark areas, 69
Benchmarking, 67
Bereavement counselor, 38
  functions of, 39
Bladder spasms, 94
Board and management of the hos-
  pice organization, 62–64

Cancer
  patients, cough in, incidence of,
    85–86
  pain associated with
  adjuvant analgesics for, 79
    common misconceptions about,
    72
Caregiver services, extended, 55
CHAP. See National League for
  Nursing Community
  Health Accreditation
  Program
Chaplain, 37
  qualifications for, 38
Constipation, 89–90
Consultants, 47–48
Continuous home care, 52–53

Continuous Quality Improvement
  (CQI), 67
  calendar, 68
Cough, incidence of, in cancer
  patients, 85–86
Counselor(s), 24, 37
  bereavement, 38
  functions of, 39
  other, 39
CQI. See Continuous Quality
  Improvement.
CRISP music therapy, 47
Cutaneous stimulation, 74

Day care, 55
Death education
  in palliative care
    problems of, 152–154
    responses to, 154–157
  for patients and families by staff,
    109–110
  points to ponder, 107
  and society, 110–111
  for staff, 108–109
Decubitus ulcers, 92–93
Delivery of hospice care, 64–65
Director, medical, hospice, 23, 32–33, 48
Drug regimen for organic intestinal
  obstruction, 89
Dyspnea, 84–85
Dysuria, 94

Emesis/anorexia/nausea, 86–88
Equipment
  for hospice care, 28
  insurance coverage of, 103
Ethics
  communication of diagnostic and
    prognostic information,
    117–118
  managing conflicting expectations
    among patients, family, and
    team, 119–120
  pain management, 118–119

Euthanasia
    definition of, 123–124
    paradigm case and two levels of
        debate on, 124
        clinical considerations of, 125
        public policy considerations of,
            125–127
Expressive therapies, 45–46
Extended caregiver services, 55

Facilities
    hospice care, 55–56, 57–59
    long-term care, 57–58
Factors affecting the role of a medical
    director, 32
Families
    death education for, 109–110
    hospice care expectations of,
        116–120
Family conferences for hospice care,
    26–27, 102–103
Fungating and ulcerating malignant
    lesions, 93

Gastrointestinal symptom manage-
    ment, 86–90
Grantwriting, general tips for, 174

Health aide, home, 41–43
Health care proxy. See Advance
    directives.
History, modern, of hospice, 3–7
Home, hospice care at, 55–56
Home care
    continuous, 52–53
    routine, 52
Home health aide, 41–43
Homemaker. See Home health aide.
Hospice(s)
    early, in the United States and
        Canada, 5–6
    historical roots of, 1–3
    Medicare certification of, 12
    modern history of, 3–7
Hospice admission criteria, 12–13
Hospice candidates, interview process
    for, 21–22
Hospice care
    current state of, 140–141
    facilities, 55–56, 57–59

family conferences for, 26–27,
    102–103
future of, 142–145
legislative role in, 6–7
levels of, 52–53
    new, 53–55
listening and answering questions
    about, 99–100
myths and misconceptions associ-
    ated with, 100
origins of, 139–140
patient, family, and team expecta-
    tions regarding, 116–120
quality of, 62–65
research
    challenges in conducting, 173–174
    design and methods of, 168–169
    future areas of, 174–175
    goals of, 168
    proposals of, 169–173
standards, 65–66
trends, 141–142
Hospice managers, 48 See hospice
    managers in Ch. 5
Hospice medical director, 23, 32–33,
    48
Hospice orientation program death
    education components, 108
Hospice patients. See Patients.
Hospice programs
    community funding for, 18
    office space and equipment needed
        for, 28
    policies in, 13
    status of, 11
Hospice services, 51
    profiles of, 13
    reimbursement for
        acceptance of patients regard-
            less of pay, 15, 18
        Medicaid, 15, 16–17
        Medicare, 14–16, 17
        private insurance, 15, 17
        Veterans Health Administration
            (VHA), 15, 17–18
Hospice staff
    and death, 111–113
    death education for, 108–109
    as interdisciplinary team members,
        48

Hospice team. See interdisciplinary team.
Hospice workers. See Interdisciplinary team.
HOSPICE WORLDWIDE, 147–148, 149–150
Hospital, 57

Inpatient care, regular, 53
Insurance
    coverage of medicines, supplies, and equipment, 103
    private, hospice benefits, 15, 17
Interdisciplinary team(s), 22–25
    in action, 26
    characteristics, 25
    conference, structure for, 27
    and home visits, 100–102
    hospice care expectations of, 116–120
    members, 41–45
        additional, 45–48
        office staff as, 48
    physician, 34
    and stress, 131–132
Intestinal obstruction, 88–89

Joint Commission on Accreditation of Health Care Organizations (JCAHO), 66

Kubler-Ross, E., 3, 5, 6

Lesions, malignant, fungating and ulcerating, 93
Living will. See Advance directives.
Long-term care facility, 57–58
Lymphedema, 94–95

Management and board of the hospice organization, 62–64
Medicaid hospice benefits, 15, 16–17
Medical director, hospice, 23, 32–33, 48
Medical social worker, 24, 36–37
Medical specialists, 47
Medicare certification of hospices, 12
Medicare hospice benefits, 14–16, 17
Medicare required facility adaptation, 56

Medications for pain management, 75–79
Medicine(s),
    insurance coverage of, 103
    palliative care, curriculum development in, 157–160
Music therapist, 46
Music therapy, CRISP, 47

National Hospice Organization (NHO), 65–66, 147–148
National League for Nursing Community Health Accreditation Program (CHAP), 66
    evaluation guidelines, 67
Nausea/emesis/anorexia, 86–88
Neurologic symptom management, 90–92
NHO. See National Hospice Organization.
Nonsteroidal anti-inflammatory drugs (NSAIDS), 75, 76–77, 78
Nurse(s), 23
    assessment, 35
    and death education in palliative care, 108
        problems regarding, 153–154
        responses to, 156–157
    on-call, 36
    and physicians, collaborative practice among, 163
    primary care, 35
    registered, 34–35
Nursing, palliative care, curriculum development in, 161–163

Obstruction, intestinal, 88–89
Occupational therapist, 44
Office Staff, 48
On Death and Dying, 5
On-call nurse, 36
Opioids, 75, 76, 77, 78, 79
Oral care for patients, 87, 88
Oxford Textbook of Palliative Medicine, 3

Pain
    assessment of, 73
    cancer associated, common misconceptions about, 72

causes of, 71–72
common misconceptions about, 72
management of, 73
    ethical dilemmas regarding,
        118–119
relief of
    nonpharmacologic approaches
        to, 74–75
    pharmacologic approaches to,
        75–79
    principles of, 74
Palliative care, 5. See also hospice care.
advance directives in, 122–123
contribution of pharmacological
    innovation to, 7–8
definition and knowledge base,
    151–152
educational programs in
    problems of, 152–154
    responses to, 154–157
legislative role in, 6–7
medicine, curriculum development
    in, 157–160
nursing, curriculum development
    in, 161–163
Patient(s)
behavioral changes in, 91–92
care plan for, 113
and death, 105–106, 111–113
death education for, 109–110
demographic information on, 14
emergencies, 103–104
general comfort measures for,
    104–105
hospice care expectations of,
    116–120
oral care for, 87, 88
profiles of, 13
Pharmacist, 45
Physical therapist, 44
Physician(s), 31
attending, 34
and death education in palliative
    care
    problems regarding, 152–153
    responses to, 155–156
interdisciplinary team, 34
and nurses, collaborative practice
    among, 163
Physician-assisted suicide. See
    Euthanasia.

Pressure sores, 92–93
Pressure ulcers, 92–93
Primary care nurse, 35
Private insurance hospice benefits,
    15, 17
Pruritus, 92
Psychosocial interventions, 75

Qualifications
    of home health aides, 42
    of a hospice medical director, 33
Quality, hospice care, 62–65

Reasons for family conferences, 103
Registered nurse, 34–35
Regular inpatient care, 53
Regulatory standards of hospice
    care, 65
Research
    challenges in conducting, 173–174
    as a component of hospice care,
        168
    components of a proposal
        data management, 173
        evaluation criteria, 170
        investigators and consultants,
            173
        literature review and theoretical
            framework, 171
        measurement, 172
        procedures, 172–173
        significance section, 171
        study aims, hypotheses, or
            study questions, 169, 171
        subjects, 172
    designs and methods of, 168–169
    future areas of, 174–175
Residences, AIDS, 59
Residential care, 54
Respirations, noisy, prior to death, 86
Respiratory symptom management,
    84–86
Respiratory therapist, 47
Respite care, 53
Responsibilities
    of a hospice medical director, 33
    of home health aides, 42
    of the interdisciplinary team, 22
    of management to provide quality
        hospice care, 64
Routine home care, 52

Saunders, C., 3–5, 6, 151–152
Seven tasks of dying, 112
Skills of home health aides, 43
Skin symptom management, 92–93
Sleeplessness, 90–91
Smith Papyrus, 7
Social worker, medical, 24, 36–37
Sources of reimbursement for hospice
    services, 15
Specialists, medical, 47
Speech therapist, 44
Stress
    coping with, through support
       groups, 133
    on hospice workers, 131–132
Suicide. See Euthanasia.
Supplies, insurance coverage of, 103
Support group(s)
    facilitators, 134–135
    membership and methodology,
       135–136
    norms for, 132–134
    techniques used in, 136
    value of, 132

TENS. See Cutaneous stimulation.
Therapist
    art, 46–47
    music, 46
    occupational, 44
    physical, 44
    respiratory, 47
    speech, 44
Therapy
    expressive, 45–46
    music, CRISP, 47
Transcutaneous electrical nerve stim-
    ulation (TENS). See Cuta-
    neous stimulation.

Ulcerating and fungating malignant
    lesions, 93
Urinary symptom management,
    93–94

Veterans Health Administration
    (VHA) hospice benefits, 15,
    17–18
Volunteers, 24, 44–45